# GORDON RAMSAY'S HEALTHY, LEAN & FIT

# GORDON RAMSAY'S HEALTHY, LEAN & FIT

Mouthwatering Recipes to Fuel You for Life

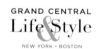

GRAND CENTRAL
Life & Style
NEW YORK · BOSTON

Copyright © 2018 by Gordon Ramsay
Photography © 2018 by Jamie Orlando Smith
Cover design by James Edgar.
Cover copyright © 2018 by Hachette Book Group, Inc.

Grand Central Life & Style
Hachette Book Group
1290 Avenue of the Americas, New York, NY 10104
grandcentrallifeandstyle.com
twitter.com/grandcentralpub

First published in Great Britain in 2018
by Hodder & Stoughton Ltd
An Hachette UK Company

First Grand Central Publishing edition: September 2018

Grand Central Life & Style is an imprint of Grand Central Publishing. The Grand Central Life & Style name and logo are trademarks of Hachette Book Group, Inc.

The Hachette Speakers Bureau provides a wide range of authors for speaking events. To find out more, go to www.hachettespeakersbureau.com or call (866) 376-6591.

Print book interior design by James Edgar.

Library of Congress Control Number: 2018938065

Cover photographs: Portrait by Victoria Wall Harris © Vanka Industries, Inc., d/b/a MasterClass; Food photography by Jamie Orlando Smith © Hodder & Stoughton, 2017; Kitchen ©Shutterstock.com

ISBNs: 978-1-5387-1466-9 (hardcover);
978-1-5387-1467-6 (ebook)

Printed in the United States of America

WOR

10  9  8  7  6  5  4  3  2  1

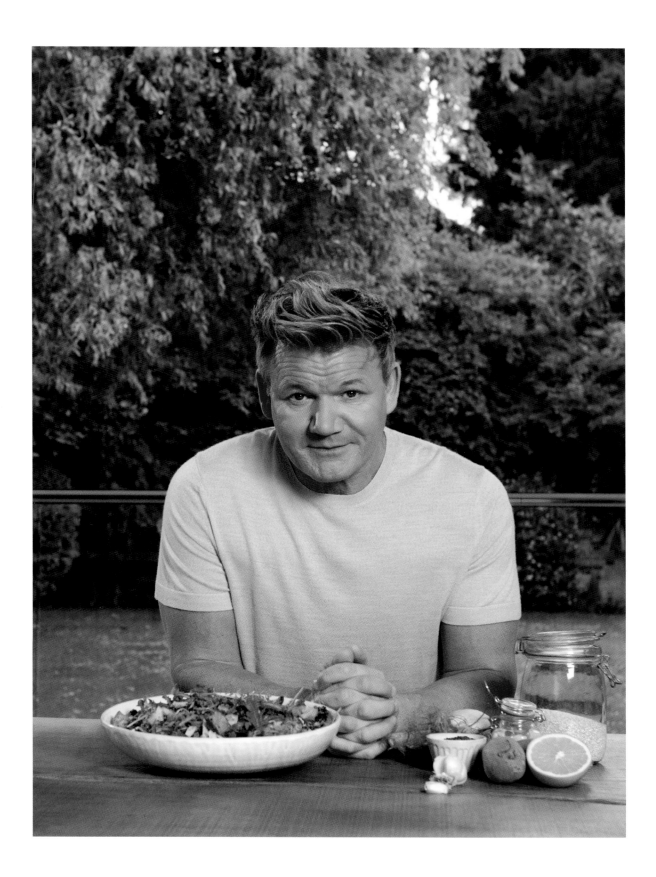

# CONTENTS

# CONTENTS

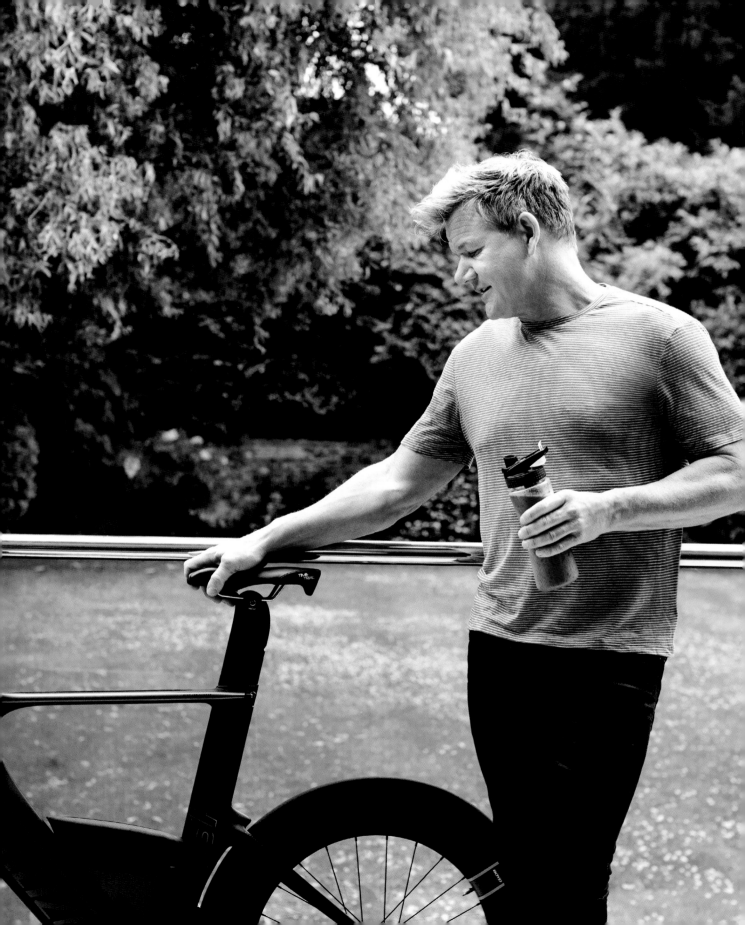

# INTRODUCTION

# I HAVE ALWAYS SAID THAT CHEFS EAT THE BEST FOOD AND THE WORST IN EQUAL MEASURE.

They work with the freshest, most delicious ingredients available, cook them perfectly, and are constantly trying little tasty mouthfuls as they work. But do they get home and make themselves a nutritious meal at the end of their sixteen-hour shift? I'm afraid they do not. The punishing working life of a chef means that they often rely on junk food and sugary snacks to get through the day, and finding time for exercise is really hard. When I was working in the restaurant at Royal Hospital Road, I never left the kitchen, sending everyone else out on their break rather than getting out myself, and I was snacking on the wrong things throughout the day. Over time, I let myself get out of shape. My chef's whites got tighter and tighter and I felt lethargic and sluggish a lot of the time.

It all changed when I started forcing myself to go to the gym for a run. I had to schedule it in like a trip to the dentist so I couldn't get out of it! I started with 5 km, then 10 km, then, before I knew it, I was running my first marathon! That was followed later the same year with an ultramarathon in South Africa . . . I was hooked. Being fit made me feel great and it became my escape from my very busy life. My eating improved, the weight came off, and I looked and felt so much better. My health improved dramatically, too. I turned fifty recently and, given that my father died of a heart attack at fifty-three, my wife, Tana, organized a complete health checkup for me. I was in training for the Ironman Triathlon World Championship in Hawaii at the time, and when they checked my pulse, it was the lowest resting heart rate for a man of my age that they had ever seen! I must be doing something right . . .

For me, being healthy involves eating well and taking exercise. This sounds obvious, but I can't stress enough the importance of doing these things in combination (though not necessarily at the same time!). To improve your diet without exercising can only get you so far when you are trying to lose weight or boost your health. Similarly, to take up exercising without considering what you eat will have only limited success. It is the combination of the two that brings better health.

But this is not a diet book telling you what (and what not) to eat, nor is it full of faddy ideas about eating cabbage soup or living off grapefruits or eating like a caveman. It works on the very simple premise that what you put into your body makes a difference in how it functions. It also acknowledges that the body has different requirements depending on what you are expecting it to do. If you are trying to lose a bit of weight, you need to eat less than when you are maintaining a healthy weight, and when you are taking part in rigorous exercise you will need to fuel your body correctly to ensure it has the resources to deliver.

Finally, healthy eating doesn't have to be dull! As a chef, I want the food that I eat to be tasty and satisfying as well as good for me. When I'm in training, I don't want my taste buds to get bored by eating the same things over and over again. And I don't ever want to feel deprived. These are my go-to recipes when I want to eat well at home, and my great hope is that they will inspire you to get cooking to improve your own health, whatever your personal goal. Here's to better health!

Gordon x

# WHAT IS HEALTHY EATING?

I am not going to get scientific here, but I do think an understanding of what the body needs and how it gets this from food can help us make better decisions when it comes to eating. I am lucky enough to have worked with personal trainers and nutritionists who have shared their knowledge with me and, once I learned the basics, making healthy decisions has become second nature.

To keep itself properly fueled and in optimum condition, the body needs a combination of macro- and micronutrients. Macronutrients are foods we need in relatively large amounts. The main three are:

**PROTEIN**—found in meat, fish, dairy products, eggs, beans, and nuts, and essential for building and repairing tissue in bones, muscles, cartilage, skin, and blood as well as for the production of hormones and important enzymes. The recommended daily intake for protein is 50 grams for women and 55 grams for men.

**CARBOHYDRATES**—the starches, sugars, and dietary fiber found in foods such as potatoes, grains (like wheat, rice, corn, etc.), beans, fruits, and vegetables that are the body's main source of energy. Fiber found in starchy carbohydrates is essential for digestive health; it helps with the elimination of waste and can prevent heart disease, some cancers, and diabetes. The recommended daily intake for carbohydrates is 260 grams for women and 300 grams for men, and health experts recommend a daily intake of roughly 30 grams of fiber for both men and women.

**FAT**—an excellent source of energy and needed for the absorption of some vital micronutrients. Confusingly, all fats are not created equal, so while the body does need some fat to survive, it is healthy unsaturated fat and not saturated fat that is required (see page 25 for more information). Fat is found in oils, animal products, fish, seeds, and nuts. The recommended daily intake of fat should be limited to 70 grams for women and 95 grams for men, of which no more than 20 grams and 30 grams, respectively, should be saturated fat.

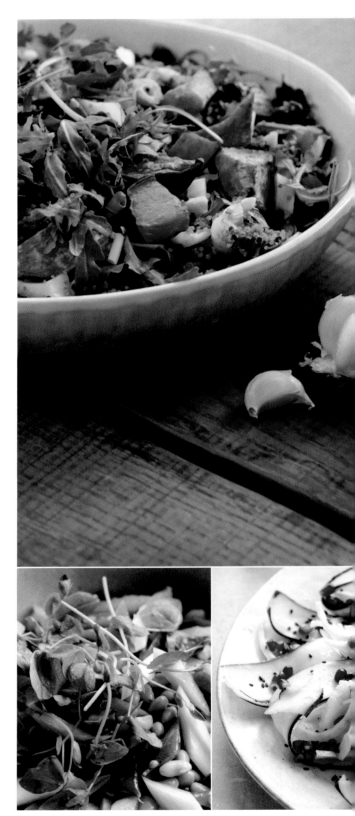

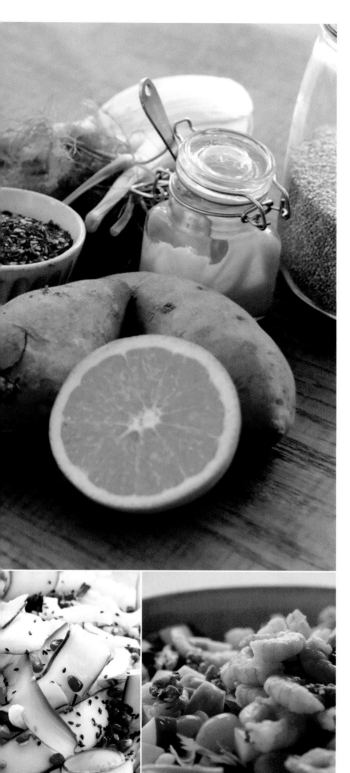

Micronutrients are the vitamins and minerals that we need in much smaller amounts but that are no less vital for normal growth and healthy development. Micronutrients include vitamins A, B complex (including folic acid), C, D, E, and K, as well as minerals like iron, calcium, magnesium, potassium, and zinc. Vitamins and minerals are found in lots of different foods, including vegetables, fruits, nuts, eggs, and dairy products, and they are important for the smooth running of our organs, eyes, skin, gut, immune system, and so on. No one food or meal contains all the vitamins and minerals we need, which is why eating a varied diet is so important.

Everything the body needs is available from the food we eat, so we should all be pretty healthy, right? Unfortunately, it isn't quite as simple as that. The problem is that there are some things that we don't need a lot of, like refined carbohydrates, saturated fat, and sugar (see page 24), but we eat lots of them because they taste good—think chips, soda, fast food, cakes, and cookies. Not only can these things be detrimental to our health when eaten in excess, if we regularly choose to fill ourselves up with the bad stuff, we are likely to be consuming too many calories and missing out on the vital nutrients and fiber present in healthier foods.

The body's requirements change if you are trying to lose weight (see page 109) and also if you lead a very active lifestyle (see page 189), but generally we should all be trying to eat as varied a diet as possible while keeping our intake of saturated fat, sugar, and salt down (see page 23). The recipes in this book will make it easy to eat the right variety of foods depending on the challenges you face.

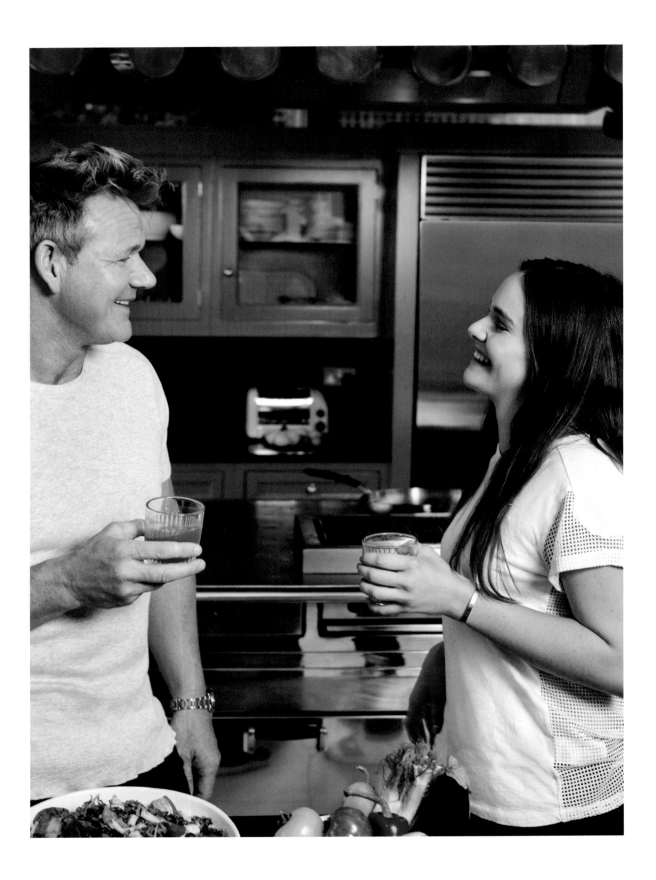

# HEALTHY KIDS

It is especially important that children get all the macro- and micronutrients that they need while they are growing and developing. The exact nutritional requirements of children and teenagers are beyond the scope of this book, but I do think that introducing kids to a wide variety of foods including plenty of fruits and vegetables from a young age helps them to develop a taste for healthy foods, and by keeping fried, processed, fatty, salty, and overly sweet foods to a minimum, you can teach them that these are treats to be indulged in only once in a while. Making smoothies, soups, and veg-packed stews and sauces is an excellent way to pack as many nutrients as possible into growing kids, even the most veg-avoiding ones, and eating together as a family can encourage your children to try new things when they see what the adults are eating.

But to me, it isn't just a case of what you feed children; it's about teaching them to make good choices and equipping them with the skills they need to look after themselves when they leave your care, skills like basic nutrition and cooking. Ever since our four children were tiny, it has been important to Tana and me that they have a good understanding of food—where it comes from, how to cook it, and how it affects our health. They are now teenagers, and it seems to have paid off. Sure, they all like pizza, chocolate, and soda like everyone else, but most of the time they eat a healthy, varied diet that balances out the special treats. They also understand the important relationship between diet and exercise and are really active. I like to think we have given them a healthy relationship with food for life.

There are lots of family-friendly recipes in this book, but it should be noted that children should not follow a low-fat diet unless instructed to by a doctor. Healthy fats are particularly vital for children's development, so restricting fat is not recommended.

# HOW TO USE
# THIS BOOK

Each of the dishes in this book has been analyzed by a nutritionist and the figures are printed alongside each recipe to help you become familiar with the nutritional content of everyday meals. These figures exclude optional items and garnishes. Based on these numbers, I have split the recipes into three sections—Healthy, Lean, and Fit.

There are no rigid rules, though. You can mix and match recipes from the different sections depending on who you are cooking for. For example, you can add a Healthy side dish to a Lean main course if you are feeding children and non-dieters, or you can serve a carbohydrate-boosting side dish from the Fit section with a Healthy supper if you are in training for a race or event. Just keep an eye on the figures over the course of a day to check that you aren't taking in more calories than you actually need.

Here are the official UK Reference Intake (RI) guidelines for moderately active men and women. These indicate what you need in a day for a healthy, balanced diet. Keep these in mind when you are planning your meals to make sure you are adequately fueling your day. You should aim not to exceed the figures listed below for fat, saturated fat, sugar, and salt. Individual needs may vary, so this should be used as a guide only.

Note that this book has been written to conform to the UK's nutritional guidelines. For US information, you can visit health.gov to view the current Dietary Guidelines for Americans, a resource that is regularly updated by the USDA and HHS.

|  | WOMEN | MEN |
|---|---|---|
| CALORIES | 2,000 | 2,500 |
| FAT (G) | 70 | 95 |
| SATURATED FAT (G) | 20 | 30 |
| CARBS (G) | 260 | 300 |
| SUGAR (G) | 90 | 120 |
| PROTEIN (G) | 50 | 55 |
| SODIUM (G) | 6 | 6 |

# HEALTHY

To be categorized as Healthy, one serving has to contain:

—no more than 5 grams of saturated fat
—no more than 15 grams of sugar
—no more than 1.5 grams of sodium per serving

These recipes are ideal for maintaining a healthy weight, keeping blood sugar levels stable, and boosting your intake of a wide variety of nutrients.

# LEAN

The dishes in the Lean section come in at:

—under 300 calories per serving for breakfast
—under 600 calories per serving for lunch and dinner
—under 150 calories for a snack

Also, a limited number of the calories are derived from fat. Choosing recipes from this section will help you to consume fewer calories, which in turn will help you to lose weight over a period of time, especially when combined with raised activity levels.

# FIT

The Fit section is full of meals and snacks that contain the right amounts, types, and combinations of macronutrients (carbohydrates, protein, and fat) for an active lifestyle. These recipes provide:

—fuel for training and endurance sports
—proteins for recovery and repairing tired muscles

There are more calories in some of these dishes to meet the needs of the body when exercising.

# NOTES ABOUT
# THE INGREDIENTS

**ANIMAL WELFARE**

Try to buy meat, eggs, and dairy products from reputable farms that value the welfare of their livestock. It isn't just better for the animals, it is better for you, as it is likely to be a more flavorful product.

**LOW-FAT FOODS**

At home, we try to eat ingredients in their most natural form so we can be sure of what we are putting into our bodies. Avoid low-fat versions of favorites because they often contain lots of sugar to make up for the lack of flavor. That said, low-fat dairy products like low-fat milk, reduced-fat coconut milk, and 0% fat Greek yogurt make it into this book when keeping fat levels down is important.

**ORGANIC INGREDIENTS**

Choose organic ingredients where you can, as they contain lower levels of pesticides and heavy metals and more nutrients. They have less impact on the environment, too, so it's a win-win.

**EGGS**

All eggs in this book are medium-size unless otherwise stated. Buy free-range eggs whenever you can.

**FISH**

Choose fish from sustainable sources, caught or farmed using environmentally friendly methods.

**OIL**

In this book, I mostly use olive, canola, and peanut oils for cooking and extra virgin olive oil for dressing, drizzling, and finishing. When choosing coconut oil, make sure it is the unrefined "virgin" variety, which is rich in a useful form of saturated fats (see page 25 for more information about coconut oil).

**HERBS**

A small bunch of herbs weighs about 1½ ounces and a large bunch weighs about 3 ounces.

**SALT**

I season my food with sea salt because it enhances the flavor, but you can leave it out if you are trying to keep your salt levels down.

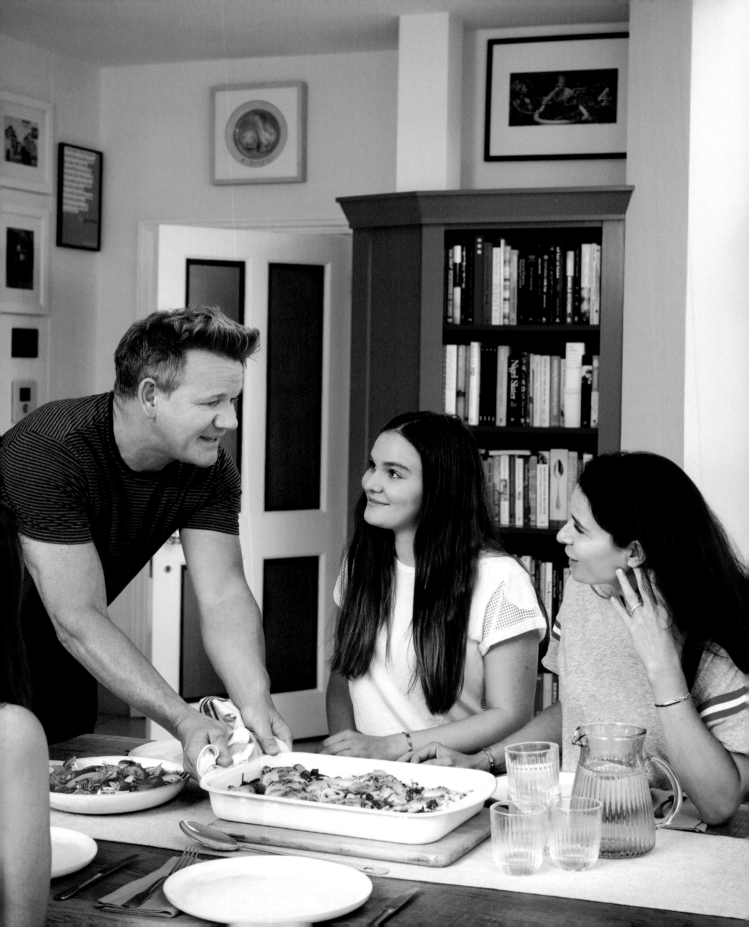

NOURISHING
BREAKFASTS

NUTRITIOUS LUNCHES
AND SALADS

SUPER SUPPERS
AND SIDES

HEALTHY SNACKS AND
NOT-TOO-SWEET TREATS

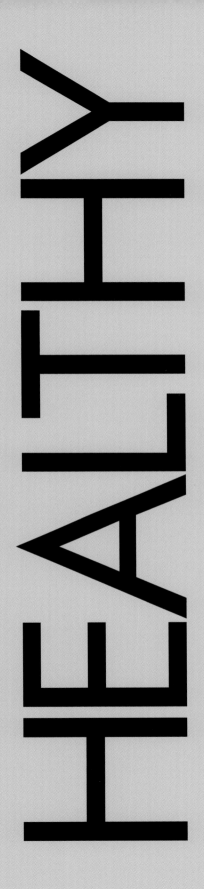

# HEALTHY

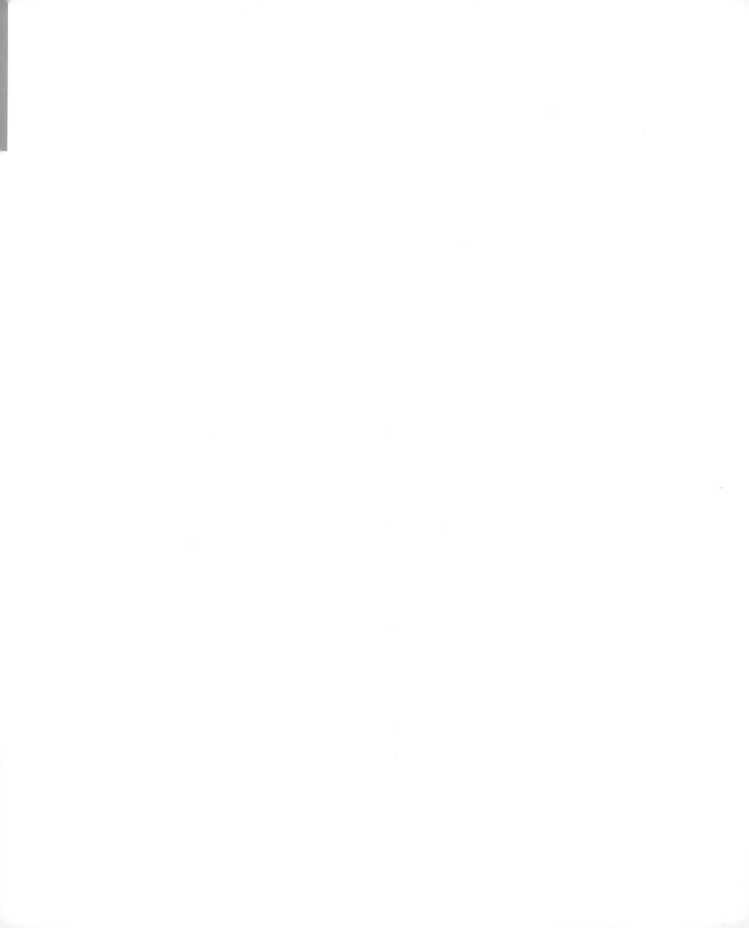

# THERE IS A LOT OF MISINFORMATION ABOUT HEALTHY EATING AROUND THESE DAYS.

It is widely agreed that consuming a diet of fried chicken, fries, cake, and cookies is not balanced or likely to be very beneficial for health! Our usual response is to try to cut down on the bad things like sugar, fat, and salt to improve our well-being. But to me, healthy eating is not just about avoiding the foods that we know are bad for us but about actively seeking out the good things and trying to eat as varied a diet as possible. This chapter is all about making good choices and finding new ways to add healthy ingredients to your meals.

One of the best ways to increase the amount and variety of nutrients and fiber in your diet is to consume more fruits and vegetables. The UK government recommends aiming to eat at least five portions every day, but recent findings suggest this number should be even higher. Happily, I love most fruits and veg, but I still need inspiration when it comes to trying new ones or finding ways to increase my daily intake. The salads, side dishes, soups, and even the snacks in this section will make hitting your five-a-day really easy.

Another way to eat your way toward better health is to ensure that you include lots of so-called superfoods in your diet. This term is controversial, because there is no official definition of a superfood, but it is generally considered to be an ingredient that punches above its weight in nutritional terms. The list includes nutrient-rich giants such as broccoli, avocados, kale, spinach, blueberries, quinoa, eggs, walnuts, and oily fish. While none of these foods have any actual magical powers, a diet that features a variety of superfoods will be very nutritious and a really positive step in the right direction.

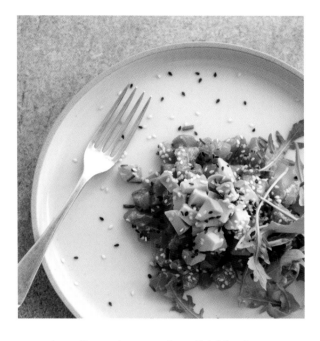

As well as eating more beneficial foods, a great way to instantly improve your health is to cook more yourself. Many people rely on the quick fix of prepared meals without realizing that they are often very high in fat, salt, and sugar, not to mention artificial colors, flavorings, emulsifiers and stabilizers, and so on. In restaurant kitchens, almost everything is made from scratch, so the food, however fancy, is actually very simple. If you cook from scratch at home, you will always know exactly what goes into your meals (and into your mouth), and you can keep the all-important fat, salt, and sugar levels down.

The great bonus of improving the quality of the food you eat is that over time you will crave the bad stuff less and less. Your tastes will start to change and you'll find healthy meals and snacks more satisfying than the greasy, sugary quick fixes you used to eat without thinking. It's a virtuous circle—the better the food you eat, the better you feel, and the better you feel, the better food choices you make, the ultimate winner being your long-term health. You just have to get started . . .

## REFINED CARBOHYDRATES AND SUGAR

When you begin to learn about nutrition, you discover that it isn't always straightforward. Take carbohydrates, for example; all carbs provide the body with energy, but it turns out that there are good and bad sources. So-called good carbs are also known as complex carbohydrates because they are relatively difficult for the body to digest, due to their chemical structure and their fiber content. They tend to be whole or unrefined and because they take longer to break down, the energy they provide is released slowly and steadily for the body to access over time. Good sources of complex carbs include whole-wheat bread, brown pasta, oats, brown rice, peas, beans, and starchy vegetables. These carbs also provide a wide range of vitamins and minerals and will make you feel fuller for longer, thanks to the dietary fiber.

"Bad" carbs, on the other hand, are known as simple carbs and are either naturally very easy to digest (e.g., sugar) or have been processed or cooked in a way that removes all the good stuff that usually slows down digestion. These refined carbs are found in white bread, white pasta, cookies, cakes, and baked goods made with white flour. The lack of dietary fiber in these foods means that the energy they provide hits the bloodstream really quickly, causing blood sugar levels to spike and crash and leaving you tired, irritable, light-headed, and hungry for more. Over time, these fluctuating sugar levels may lead to weight gain, which can increase your risk of developing health problems like heart disease and possibly diabetes.

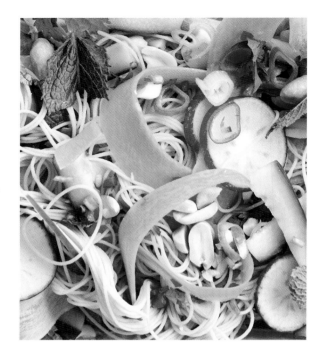

Because nutrition isn't straightforward, there are two types of sugar, too. Naturally occurring sugars are found in fruits, vegetables, and dairy products and are not considered a problem for health as long as they are eaten in the form that nature intended; in fact, they can be an excellent source of accessible energy. But the other type, known as "free" sugar, is definitely considered a problem. Free sugars include those that are added to our food, like regular sugar, white and brown, as well as other sweeteners such as honey, maple syrup, corn syrup, palm sugar, agave syrup, and fruit juices. It is these sugars that we are advised to cut down on, because they provide lots of calories without much or any goodness and we tend to consume too much of them, not least because they are often hidden in prepared meals, snacks, and soda to make them taste better. Consuming too much sugar is one of the major causes of obesity and tooth decay around the world, and cutting back is a really positive way to improve your health. The recipes in this book do include free sugars such as honey, maple syrup, and agave syrup, but in small quantities and combined with complex carbohydrates and sometimes protein to slow down their effect.

## FAT

Fat has had a hard time over the years. It's been blamed for obesity, raised cholesterol levels, and heart disease, and we have been told to keep our intake to a minimum. But like many pieces of nutritional advice, the reality is not so simple; it turns out we actually need some fat in our diet to stay healthy. It's a valuable source of energy and is essential for the absorption of various important vitamins like A, D, E, and K and for the production of hormones.

Like sugar and carbs, there are two main types of fat and, historically, saturated fat found in animal products like lard, butter, and cheese has been considered "bad" fat, while unsaturated fats from plant sources like olive, sunflower, and nut oils, as well as oily fish, is thought of as "good" fat. But a number of recent studies are questioning these long-held beliefs and are suggesting that saturated fat isn't quite as bad for us as previously thought. While this may be good news for those of us who enjoy a nicely marbled steak and cooking with butter from time to time, the government guidelines haven't changed, and we are still advised to keep our intake of saturated fat to below 20 grams a day for women and 30 grams for men.

Some of the recipes in this book use coconut oil, which is worth mentioning here because although it comes from a plant, it actually contains a lot of saturated fat—but it's a special type of saturated fat that is thought to be helpful for weight loss by both reducing appetite and boosting metabolism. When buying coconut oil, choose the unrefined virgin variety because it is rich in these special fats.

There are also other forms of fat that are critical to good health; these essential fats (known as omega-3s) are good for your heart and important for learning and behavior. Good sources include oily fish like salmon and trout and, to a lesser extent, nuts and seeds like walnuts, chia seeds, and flaxseeds, and we should actively try to consume more of them.

Whether the fat comes from saturated or unsaturated sources, the key thing to remember is that fat provides, gram for gram, over twice as much energy as carbohydrates and protein. So if you are consuming too much fat without burning it off through exercise, the excess energy will be stored as body fat. Whatever the recent findings about fat being good for you, it is no time to celebrate with a plate of fish and chips!

## A WORD ABOUT HYDRATION

Almost more important than what you eat is how much you drink. A human being can survive more than three weeks without eating but would die after three days without water. At least 60 percent of the body is water, and it is vital to keep liquid levels topped off throughout the day, particularly if you are exercising (see page 191 for more information about hydrating for sports). It is recommended that we drink 6 to 8 glasses of water a day to ward off dehydration, which can give you a headache and make you feel irritable and drowsy. Happily, other drinks such as coffee, tea, milk, fruit juice, and smoothies all count toward your liquid intake over the day. On top of this, about 20 percent of the fluid we consume comes from the food that we eat, especially if we eat lots of fruits and vegetables—another reason to aim to beat our five-a-day target.

# NOURISHING BREAKFASTS

# APPLE, MINT, SPINACH, LIME, AND CUCUMBER JUICE

**SERVES 2**

A freshly squeezed juice is a great, vitamin-packed way to start the day. It wakes up the taste buds and rehydrates the body after a long night's sleep. Juices count as one of your five-a-day, so you'll be getting off to a racing start before you have even eaten your breakfast. This is particularly good for getting kids to eat spinach because they won't be able to taste it. You could also serve it on ice as a really refreshing mocktail for summer entertaining.

1 green apple, cored and quartered
4 mint sprigs, leaves only
2 big handfuls of spinach leaves, washed
Juice of 1½ limes
½ cucumber, roughly chopped

**1**. Pass all the ingredients through a juicer or combine them in a blender and blend until smooth. If the mixture needs help going through a juicer, add a little cold water as you juice.

**2**. Serve in a tall glass with ice.

| PER SERVING | |
|---|---|
| CALORIES | 48 |
| FAT (g) | 1.0 |
| SATURATED FAT (g) | 0.1 |
| CARBS (g) | 7.0 |
| SUGAR (g) | 7.0 |
| FIBER (g) | 1.0 |
| PROTEIN (g) | 2.0 |
| SODIUM (g) | 0.03 |

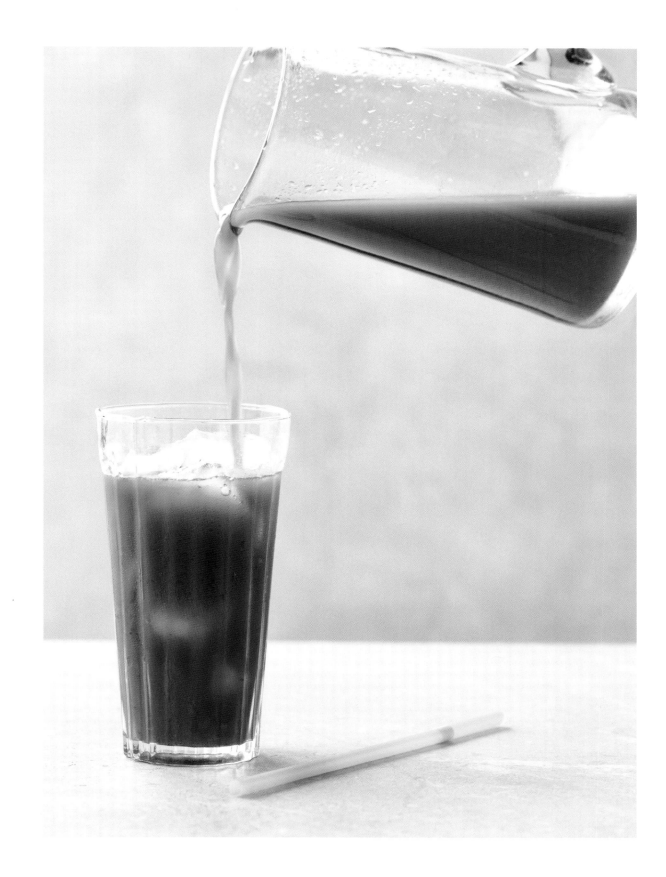

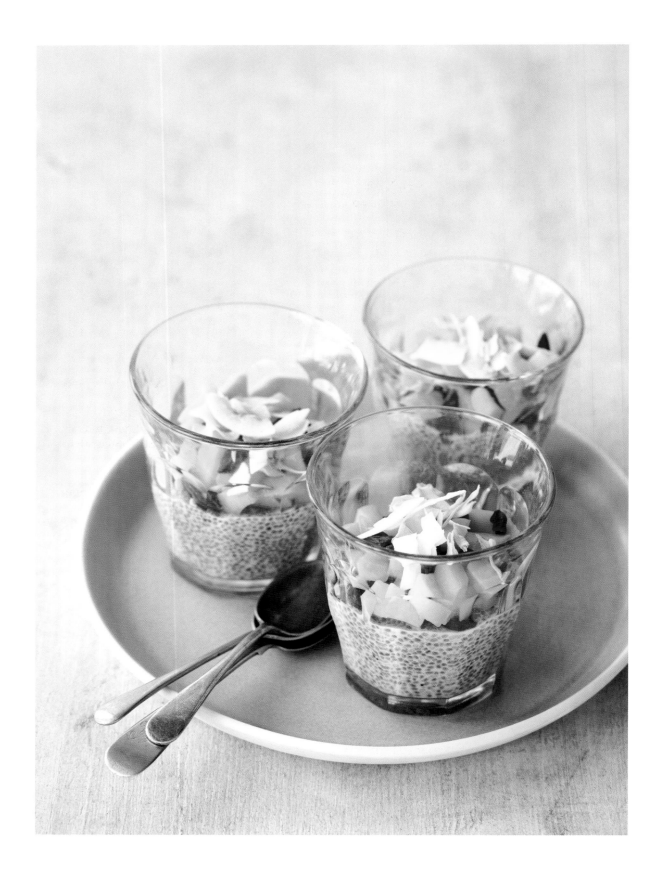

# TROPICAL CHIA
# SEED PUDDING
**SERVES 4**

My wife, Tana, introduced me to this very
fashionable, light breakfast. She's a really healthy
eater and gets the rest of us to eat our greens and
try new things like chia seeds, coconut water, and
goji berries. Chia seeds are full of good things like
plant protein, fiber, antioxidants, omega-3 fatty
acids, and minerals, but they're not just really good
for you, they're also really clever—they can absorb
approximately ten times their own weight in liquid,
which is how they are magically turned into these
delicious breakfast bowls.

2 cups coconut milk beverage
½ cup chia seeds
½ teaspoon vanilla extract
1 mango, diced
2 tablespoons goji berries
2 tablespoons toasted coconut flakes (optional)

**1**. Pour the coconut milk into a liquid measuring cup.

**2**. Divide the chia seeds among four bowls or glasses
and add one quarter of the coconut milk and one
quarter of the vanilla extract to each bowl. Stir to
combine.

**3**. Cover and place in the fridge for at least 1 hour
or overnight.

**4**. Once ready to eat, put the diced mango and goji
berries on top of the chia seeds and sprinkle over the
toasted coconut, if using.

**VARIATIONS**
Chia seed pudding can also be made with other
milks, such as almond, rice, soy, oat, or cow's,
and topped with different fruits, nuts, and seeds,
so experiment with flavors that you like—just
remember the basic ratio of one part chia seeds
to four parts liquid.

| PER SERVING | |
| --- | --- |
| CALORIES | 230 |
| FAT (g) | 13.0 |
| SATURATED FAT (g) | 3.5 |
| CARBS (g) | 27.0 |
| SUGAR (g) | 13.0 |
| FIBER (g) | 14.0 |
| PROTEIN (g) | 7.0 |
| SODIUM (g) | 0.17 |

# RASPBERRY CHIA SEED JAM

**MAKES 1 PINT**

This is the quickest, easiest, and healthiest jam recipe around. It uses the gelling power of chia seeds to transform raspberries into jam without having to worry about special pans, thermometers, or pectin. And it's good for you, too! The amount of honey will depend on the ripeness of the raspberries, so taste as you go.

8 ounces (2 cups) fresh raspberries (see below)
Juice of ½ lemon
2 to 3 tablespoons runny honey, to taste
3 tablespoons chia seeds

**1.** Put the raspberries and lemon juice into a blender with 2 tablespoons of the honey and blitz until smooth. Taste and add a little more honey if necessary.

**2.** Add the chia seeds and briefly blitz again to mix.

**3.** Transfer to a clean pint jar with a lid and allow to set in the fridge for 1 hour. This will keep for a few days in the fridge.

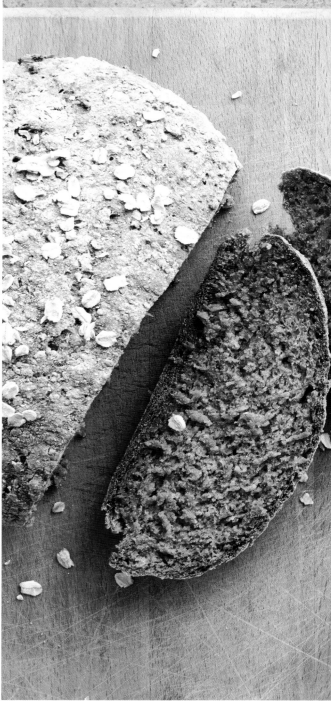

| PER TABLESPOON | |
| --- | --- |
| CALORIES | 17 |
| FAT (g) | 1.0 |
| SATURATED FAT (g) | 0.1 |
| CARBS (g) | 1.0 |
| SUGAR (g) | 1.0 |
| FIBER (g) | 1.0 |
| PROTEIN (g) | 0.5 |
| SODIUM (g) | 0.0 |

**VARIATION**
You can also use frozen raspberries for this recipe, which means you can make delicious jam all year round. Defrost the fruit slightly before blitzing.

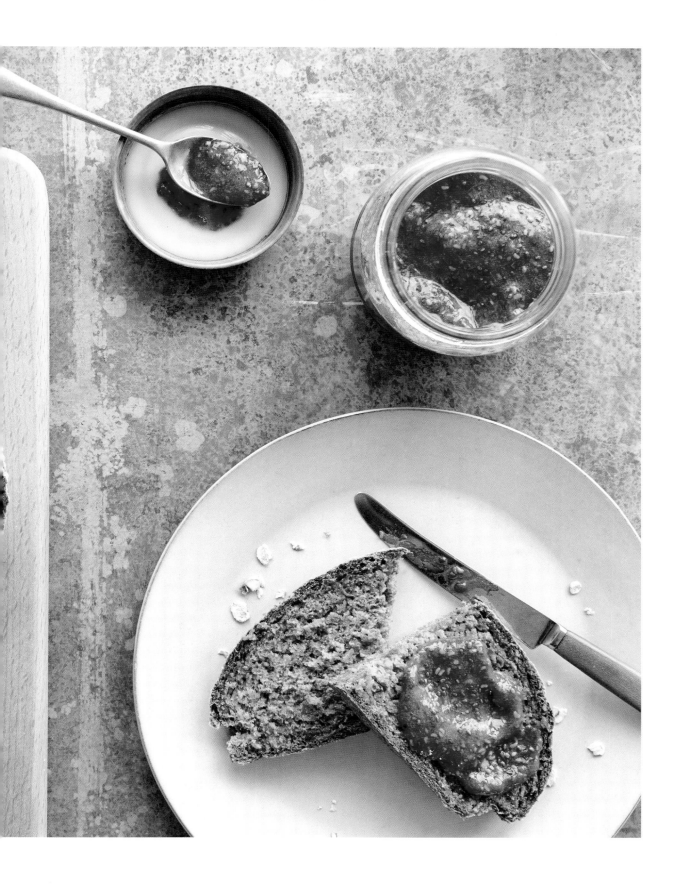

# TOASTED OAT SODA BREAD

**MAKES 1 LARGE LOAF (ROUGHLY 12 SLICES)**

If you have never baked bread before, a traditional Irish soda bread is a good place to start. It is "raised" with baking soda rather than yeast, so there is no need to wait around for it to proof, and it's pretty difficult for it to go wrong. Toasting the oats before adding them gives them a darker color and nutty flavor that works really well here. It is especially delicious toasted and served with the Raspberry Chia Seed Jam on page 32.

1⅛ cups rolled oats, plus extra for scattering over the surface
1 cup boiling water
Neutral oil, such as peanut, for greasing
¾ cup buttermilk, plus a little extra for brushing (see below)
⅔ cup skim milk
2 teaspoons baking soda
3 cups whole-wheat flour
1 teaspoon fine sea salt

**1.** Preheat the oven to 400°F.

**2.** Scatter the oats over a baking sheet and bake in the oven for about 10 minutes, turning occasionally. The oats should become nutty and dark in color.

**3.** Tip the browned oats straight into a large bowl and pour the boiling water over. Leave the oats to soak until cooled completely, about 30 minutes.

**4.** Meanwhile, reduce the oven temperature to 350°F and grease the pan you toasted the oats in.

**5.** Add the buttermilk and milk to the oats and water, then beat until thoroughly incorporated. Mix the baking soda, flour, and salt in a separate bowl. Add the wet ingredients to the dry and mix to combine.

**6.** Using floured hands, shape the dough into a ball. Transfer to the prepared pan and flatten slightly. Place in the oven and bake for 20 minutes. Quickly remove from the oven, brush with a little buttermilk, then scatter a small handful of oats over and return to the oven for an additional 30 minutes, or until browned and a tester inserted into the center comes out clean. If the bread is coloring too much, cover with aluminum foil for the remaining time.

**7.** Leave the bread to cool completely in the pan, then serve.

| PER SLICE | |
|---|---|
| CALORIES | 171 |
| FAT (g) | 2.0 |
| SATURATED FAT (g) | 0.3 |
| CARBS (g) | 31.0 |
| SUGAR (g) | 2.0 |
| FIBER (g) | 4.0 |
| PROTEIN (g) | 6.0 |
| SODIUM (g) | 0.90 |

**VARIATION**
If you can't buy buttermilk, use regular milk instead, but add a level teaspoon of cream of tartar with the baking soda.

# OAT AND QUINOA PORRIDGE WITH MIXED SEEDS

**SERVES 4**

Being Scottish, I eat porridge for breakfast all the time. I must know over a hundred different ways of serving it! This version has added quinoa, which gives it a bit of crunch and makes it a source of complete protein, extra fiber, and energizing B vitamins. Topping it off with berries and mixed seeds makes it the healthiest porridge I know.

Sea salt
1 cup quinoa, rinsed
½ cup old-fashioned rolled oats
7 ounces fresh berries, such as raspberries, blackberries, strawberries, and blueberries
¼ cup mixed seeds, such as sunflower, pumpkin, and flaxseeds
Maple syrup, to taste

**1**. Bring 1 quart of water with a pinch of salt to a simmer in a heavy-bottomed saucepan. Once simmering, stir in the quinoa and cook gently for 10 minutes, stirring occasionally.

**2**. Add the oats and stir. Continue to simmer for an additional 10 minutes, or until thick and porridge-like.

**3**. Remove the pan from the heat and divide the porridge among serving bowls. Top with the berries, sprinkle over the seeds, and drizzle with a little maple syrup for extra sweetness. Serve immediately.

**HOW TO MAKE AHEAD**
To speed things up in the morning, pre-cook the quinoa and soak overnight with the oats, so all you need to do is heat it through the next morning. Just reduce the amount of liquid you use to cook the porridge by ¾ cup.

| PER SERVING | |
| --- | --- |
| CALORIES | 315 |
| FAT (g) | 10.0 |
| SATURATED FAT (g) | 1.0 |
| CARBS (g) | 40.0 |
| SUGAR (g) | 5.0 |
| FIBER (g) | 8.0 |
| PROTEIN (g) | 12.0 |
| SODIUM (g) | 0.20 |

# APPLE PIE–SPICED OATMEAL

**SERVES 4**

This is another of my favorite oatmeal recipes, this time flavored with apple pie spices and sweetened with apples and dates, which goes down really well with the junior members of my family—it tastes like dessert! It's especially warming and delicious and the perfect thing to get you out of bed on a cold winter's morning. And with its slow-releasing energy, it should keep you going until lunchtime.

2 cups old-fashioned rolled oats
4 dates, pitted and finely chopped
½ teaspoon ground cinnamon
Pinch of freshly grated nutmeg
Pinch of ground allspice
2 apples, cored and cut into chunks
Sea salt
1¾ cups 2% low-fat milk, plus extra to serve

1. Put the oats, chopped dates, and spices into a medium heavy-bottomed saucepan with three-quarters of the apple chunks and add a pinch of salt. Pour in the milk and 1¾ cups of hot water and stir over medium heat until the porridge begins to simmer.

2. Simmer gently for 15 to 20 minutes, stirring regularly for a creamy consistency. The apple chunks will collapse into the oatmeal and the liquid should all be absorbed.

3. To serve, spoon into warmed bowls and top with the remaining apple chunks. Serve with a little pitcher of extra milk on the side.

| PER SERVING | |
| --- | --- |
| CALORIES | 231 |
| FAT (g) | 5.0 |
| SATURATED FAT (g) | 2.0 |
| CARBS (g) | 36.0 |
| SUGAR (g) | 15.0 |
| FIBER (g) | 4.0 |
| PROTEIN (g) | 8.0 |
| SODIUM (g) | 0.23 |

**VARIATIONS**
Swap the cow's milk for soy, rice, or oat milk, or, for a very lean version, make it just with water.

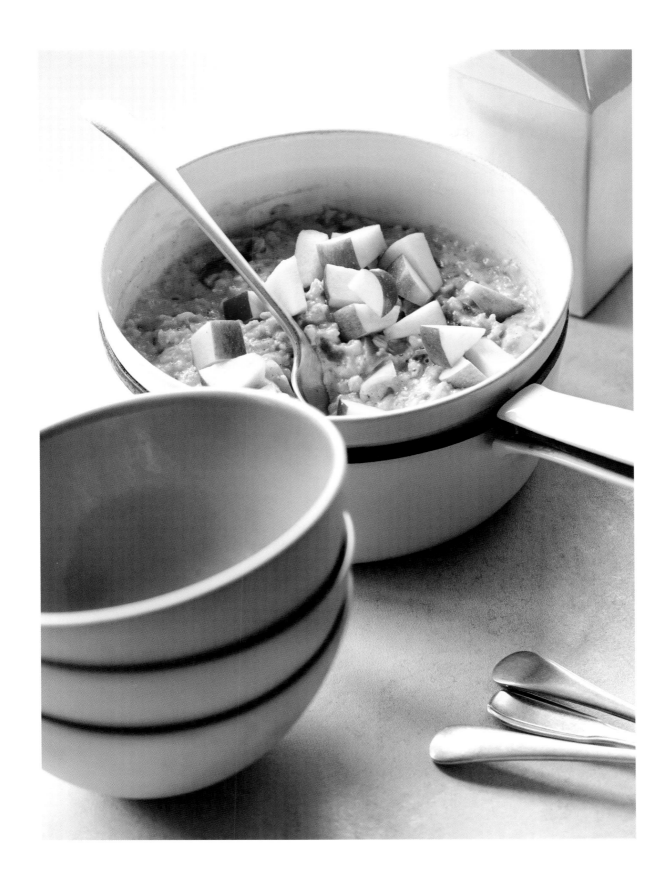

# RAINBOW VEGETABLE FRITTATA

**SERVES 4**

Cooking breakfast for the family can be a bit hectic in the morning, with everyone wanting different things, but making a frittata is much less labor-intensive while still satisfying the desire for something hot. It's better for you, too—this version is full of healthy veg to get the day off to a good start and, thanks to the protein-rich eggs, would make an ideal post-run brunch. Serve it straight from the broiler or at room temperature.

Olive oil
2 garlic cloves, peeled and finely chopped
1 red pepper, seeded and sliced
1 orange pepper, seeded and sliced
Sea salt
1 zucchini, cut into small chunks
5 stalks rainbow chard, thinly sliced
8 eggs, beaten
Freshly ground black pepper

1. Preheat the broiler.

2. Heat a dash of oil in a 10-inch nonstick, ovenproof skillet over medium heat. Add the garlic and cook until just cooked through but not turning golden.

3. Add the bell peppers and a pinch of salt and sauté for 5 to 6 minutes, until softened. Add the zucchini and cook for 2 minutes to soften slightly, then add the chard along with 1 tablespoon of hot water (if using spinach, there is no need to add the hot water) and continue to cook for 4 to 5 minutes, stirring gently, until the chard has wilted.

4. Season the beaten eggs with salt and pepper and pour over the vegetables, gently shaking the pan to make sure they are evenly spread out. Cook over medium-low heat for 5 to 7 minutes, until the frittata is almost set. Transfer to the broiler for a couple of minutes, until the top is golden and the frittata is cooked through.

5. Remove from the broiler and loosen the edges of the frittata from the pan. Slide onto a serving board or plate and cut into wedges to serve.

| PER SERVING | |
| --- | --- |
| CALORIES | 203 |
| FAT (g) | 11.0 |
| SATURATED FAT (g) | 3.0 |
| CARBS (g) | 6.0 |
| SUGAR (g) | 5.0 |
| FIBER (g) | 3.0 |
| PROTEIN (g) | 17.0 |
| SODIUM (g) | 0.76 |

**VARIATION**

If you can't get hold of rainbow chard, replace it with a handful of Swiss chard, spinach, or another green leafy vegetable, such as spring greens or kale, though these will take longer to soften.

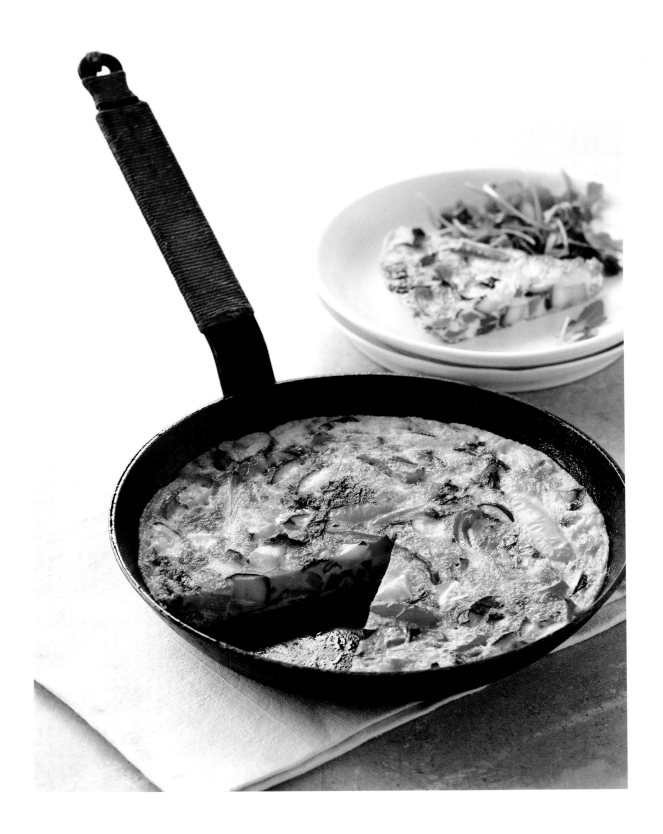

# NUTRITIOUS LUNCHES AND SALADS

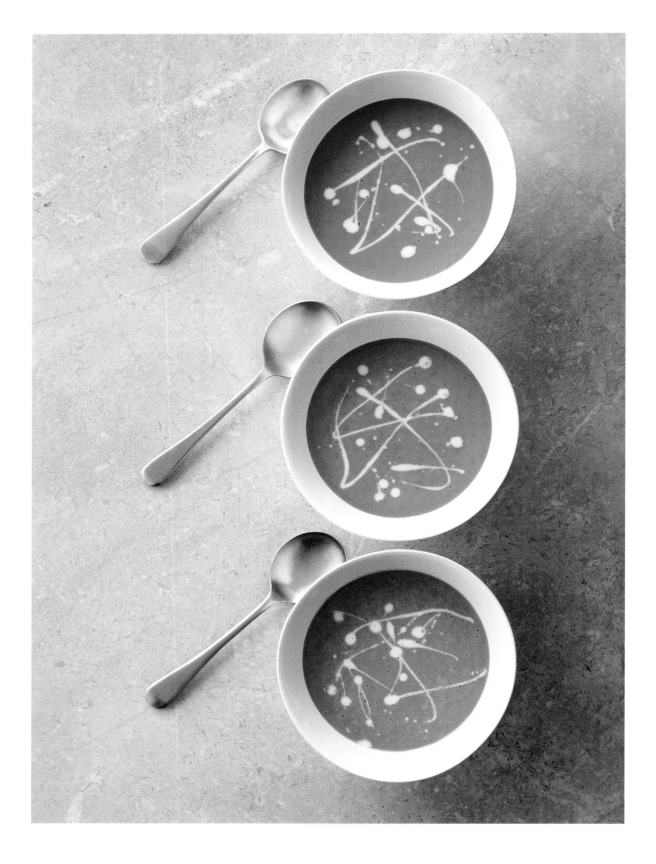

# CHILLED PEA AND COCONUT SOUP
**SERVES 6**

I think that a chilled soup is a very elegant dish to serve at a summer lunch or in shot glasses as a canapé, and this one is really easy to make while still being packed full of flavor and richness, not to mention goodness. If the weather doesn't go your way, it's also good heated up. Coconut milk does contain a lot of saturated fat, so keep an eye on portion sizes here or serve it when you know you are going to be active to use up all the easily metabolized energy it provides (see page 189).

1 (13.5-ounce) can reduced-fat coconut milk
1¾ cups coconut water
Juice of 1 lemon
3⅓ cups spinach leaves, washed
½ bunch of mint, leaves roughly chopped
5 cups frozen peas, defrosted
1-inch piece of fresh ginger, peeled and
   roughly chopped
1 green chile, seeded and roughly chopped
Sea salt and freshly ground black pepper

**1.** Set aside 3 tablespoons of the coconut milk, then put the rest of the ingredients into a blender with 2½ cups of water. Add a couple of pinches of salt and pepper and blend until really smooth. Depending on the size of your blender, you may need to do this in batches. If this is the case, divide the ingredients in half and blend together.

**2.** Taste the soup and adjust the seasoning if necessary.

**3.** Stir before serving, and serve chilled, drizzled with the reserved coconut milk.

**HOW TO SERVE IT WARM**
As the flavors in chilled soup can be a little muted, be generous with the seasoning and taste often. On the flip side, if you are serving this soup warm, watch the chile levels—the effects will be stronger, so add less if you don't like things too hot.

| PER SERVING | |
| --- | --- |
| CALORIES | 117 |
| FAT (g) | 6.0 |
| SATURATED FAT(g) | 5.0 |
| CARBS (g) | 17.0 |
| SUGAR (g) | 9.0 |
| FIBER (g) | 8.0 |
| PROTEIN (g) | 9.0 |
| SODIUM (g) | 0.21 |

# CORONATION CHICKPEAS

**SERVES 4**

Chickpeas carry spice brilliantly, so they are the base of this vegetarian take on coronation chicken. Unlike the classic cold chicken dish, this is not drenched in mayonnaise but is made healthier with a yogurt-based dressing, and you won't miss the chicken because chickpeas are rich in fiber, which helps fill you up, regulates appetite, and reduces cravings. This salad is almost better if you make it in advance, as the flavors really get a chance to meld together, so make it the day before you eat it if you can. Serve with cooled basmati rice and a crisp green salad to make a meal of it.

2 (15-ounce) cans chickpeas, drained and rinsed
1 small cauliflower, cut into really small florets
2 carrots, diced
3 spring onions, trimmed and finely chopped

**FOR THE DRESSING**
¾ cup plain yogurt
2 teaspoons curry powder
½ teaspoon ground turmeric
1 teaspoon ground cumin
2 teaspoons cider vinegar
1 teaspoon Dijon mustard
Sea salt and freshly ground black pepper

1. Put the drained chickpeas, cauliflower florets, carrots, and spring onions into a large bowl and toss to mix.

2. In a smaller bowl, mix together the dressing ingredients and season with salt and pepper.

3. Pour the dressing over the chickpeas and mix really well so that everything is coated. Taste and adjust the seasoning if necessary. Cover and store in the fridge until ready to use. It will last for up to 3 days in the fridge.

| PER SERVING | |
| --- | --- |
| CALORIES | 243 |
| FAT (g) | 6.0 |
| SATURATED FAT (g) | 1.0 |
| CARBS (g) | 29.0 |
| SUGAR (g) | 9.0 |
| FIBER (g) | 10.0 |
| PROTEIN (g) | 14.0 |
| SODIUM (g) | 0.31 |

# ROASTED BUTTERNUT SQUASH, FARRO, AND SUMAC SALAD

**SERVES 4**

Sumac is a citrusy spice that is popular in the Middle East. It lifts the earthy flavors of this salad, counterbalancing the sweetness of the butternut squash and giving the dish a lemony freshness. It's a great addition to your pantry and goes brilliantly wherever you might add a squeeze of lemon. Farro is a grain similar to pearl barley that is nutty and chewy when cooked. Though wheat has gotten a bad name for itself in these gluten-fearing times, these unprocessed whole grains are an excellent source of fiber, protein, and energizing B vitamins, and they turn this salad into a substantial meal.

1 large butternut squash, peeled, halved lengthwise, and seeded
4 garlic cloves, smashed but not peeled
Olive oil, for drizzling
Sea salt and freshly ground black pepper
1 teaspoon sumac, plus extra for sprinkling
1 cup farro
1½ cups chopped (bite-size pieces) kale
¼ cup slivered almonds, toasted, to serve

**FOR THE DRESSING**
Juice of 1 lemon
2 tablespoons tahini
½ teaspoon sumac
½ teaspoon runny honey
Pinch of sea salt and freshly ground black pepper

**CONTINUED ON PAGE 47**

| PER SERVING | |
| --- | --- |
| CALORIES | 367 |
| FAT (g) | 13.0 |
| SATURATED FAT (g) | 2.0 |
| CARBS (g) | 43.0 |
| SUGAR (g) | 11.0 |
| FIBER (g) | 10.0 |
| PROTEIN (g) | 14.0 |
| SODIUM (g) | 0.05 |

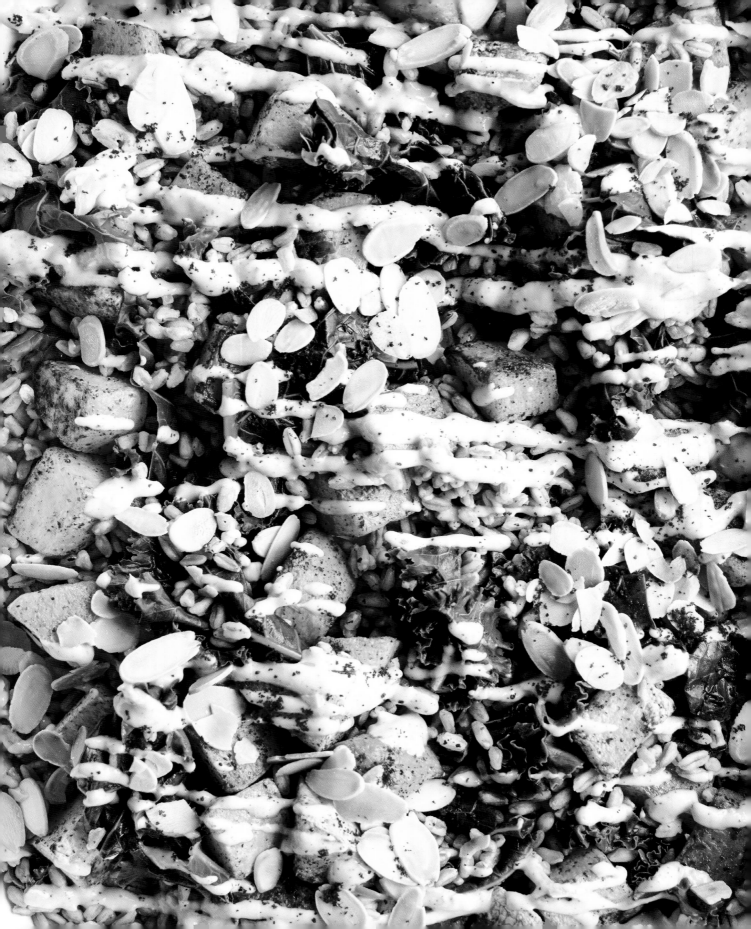

CONTINUED FROM PAGE 45

1. Preheat the oven to 400°F.

2. Cut the butternut squash into ¾-inch cubes. Put them into a roasting pan with the smashed garlic cloves and drizzle with a little olive oil. Season with salt and pepper and sprinkle over the sumac. Toss to coat evenly, then place in the oven and roast for 30 to 35 minutes, until softened and lightly browned on the edges.

3. Meanwhile, bring a pot of water to a boil and add the farro. Simmer over medium–low heat for 20 to 30 minutes, until the farro is tender but not soft. For the last 5 minutes of the cooking time, add the kale to the pan and stir through.

4. Once the kale and farro are cooked, remove from the heat, drain, and leave to cool.

5. When the butternut squash is ready, remove the pan from the oven. Pick out the garlic and squeeze the flesh out of the skins into a small mixing bowl. Mash the garlic with the back of a fork and add the dressing ingredients with a pinch of salt and pepper. Mix together really well with a fork to combine, then drizzle in 1 tablespoon of water, stirring continuously.

6. Put the farro, kale, and butternut squash into a large serving bowl and toss gently to mix together. Drizzle over the dressing and sprinkle with the almonds and a little extra sumac. Serve immediately or store in the fridge for up to 4 days. Toss well before serving.

**VARIATIONS**
You can substitute pumpkin, sweet potatoes, or carrots for the butternut squash. And if you can't get ahold of farro, it can be replaced with spelt, freekeh, or bulgur wheat. This salad would also be delicious with the addition of spoonfuls of ricotta or goat cheese dotted on top.

# ROASTED CAULIFLOWER, QUINOA, AND POMEGRANATE SALAD

**SERVES 4**

Roasting brassicas like cauliflower, broccoli, kale, and cabbage intensifies the flavor and they become sweet and almost caramelized around the edges. Cooking cauliflower this way and tossing it in this sharp pomegranate molasses dressing might just convert a few cauliflower haters to the cause. It's a vibrant, satisfying salad that works really well with slow-cooked lamb, grilled chicken, or halloumi.

1 large cauliflower, cut into florets
Olive oil, for drizzling
Sea salt and freshly ground black pepper
1 cup quinoa, rinsed
Small bunch of flat-leaf parsley, leaves picked
Seeds from 1 pomegranate, to serve

**FOR THE DRESSING**
1 tablespoon pomegranate molasses
1 tablespoon white wine vinegar
1 garlic clove, peeled and crushed
6 tablespoons extra virgin olive oil
Sea salt and freshly ground black pepper

1. Preheat the oven to 375°F.

2. Place the cauliflower florets on a baking sheet and drizzle with a little olive oil. Season with salt and pepper and toss in the oil to coat. Transfer to the oven and roast for about 20 minutes, turning the cauliflower halfway through, until browned in places. Remove from the oven once cooked.

3. Meanwhile, cook the quinoa according to the package instructions.

4. Using a small whisk or a fork, mix the ingredients for the dressing together with a pinch of salt and pepper until completely combined. Taste and adjust the seasoning if necessary.

5. Put the cooked quinoa and the cauliflower into a large bowl. Drizzle with the dressing and fold in the parsley leaves. Scatter over the pomegranate seeds and serve.

| PER SERVING | |
|---|---|
| CALORIES | 386 |
| FAT (g) | 21.0 |
| SATURATED FAT (g) | 3.0 |
| CARBS (g) | 36.0 |
| SUGAR (g) | 10.0 |
| FIBER (g) | 7.0 |
| PROTEIN (g) | 11.0 |
| SODIUM (g) | 0.11 |

**GOOD TO KNOW**
Pomegranate seeds are bursting with vitamin C, which boosts your immune system, and vitamin K, which is essential for bone and blood health. In addition to fighting bacteria, supporting the heart, and lowering blood pressure, they are also supposed to be aphrodisiacs!

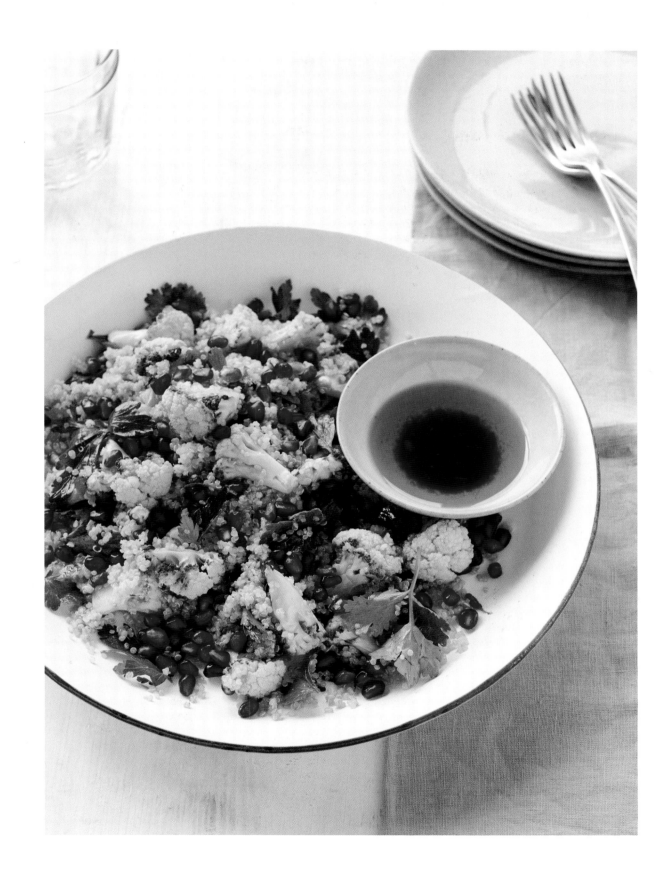

# ADZUKI BEAN, SWEET POTATO, AND FENNEL SALAD

**SERVES 4**

This is my kind of salad—it's substantial and tasty and has a great combination of earthy colors and flavors. Furthermore, thanks to the protein in the beans and quinoa, it will fill you up for the rest of the afternoon. It's delicious served warm but is just as good cold, so it can be made in advance or even the night before.

2 medium sweet potatoes, scrubbed clean and cubed
Olive oil
Sea salt and freshly ground black pepper
3 cups chopped (bite-size pieces) kale leaves
1 garlic clove, peeled and finely chopped
2 ounces (3 cups) arugula
1 (15-ounce) can adzuki beans, drained and rinsed
1⅓ cups cooked quinoa (from approximately ½ cup uncooked quinoa)
1 large fennel bulb, diced, to serve

**FOR THE DRESSING**
1 garlic clove, peeled and crushed
1½ tablespoons cider vinegar
1 heaping teaspoon Dijon mustard
Juice of ½ orange
½ teaspoon dried chile flakes (optional)
Sea salt and freshly ground black pepper
4½ tablespoons extra virgin olive oil

1. Preheat the oven to 350°F.

2. Toss the cubed sweet potatoes in a little oil and season with salt and pepper. Spread in a single layer on a baking sheet, place in the oven, and bake for 30 minutes, turning halfway through.

3. Meanwhile, place a large skillet over medium heat and add a dash of oil. When hot, add the kale with a pinch of salt and 2 tablespoons of water. Sauté for 2 minutes, or until the kale has wilted and the water has evaporated. Add the garlic and stir through. Continue to cook for an additional 2 minutes, or until the garlic has softened.

4. To make the dressing, in a large salad bowl, whisk together the garlic, vinegar, mustard, orange juice, and chile flakes, if using. Season with a pinch of salt and pepper, then slowly pour in the olive oil, whisking continuously until emulsified. Taste and adjust the flavors as necessary.

5. Put the arugula into the bowl, then add the adzuki beans, quinoa, roasted sweet potatoes, and kale and gently mix together. Scatter over the diced fennel and serve.

| PER SERVING | |
|---|---|
| CALORIES | 447 |
| FAT (g) | 16.0 |
| SATURATED FAT (g) | 2.0 |
| CARBS (g) | 55.0 |
| SUGAR (g) | 15.0 |
| FIBER (g) | 13.0 |
| PROTEIN (g) | 13.0 |
| SODIUM (g) | 0.36 |

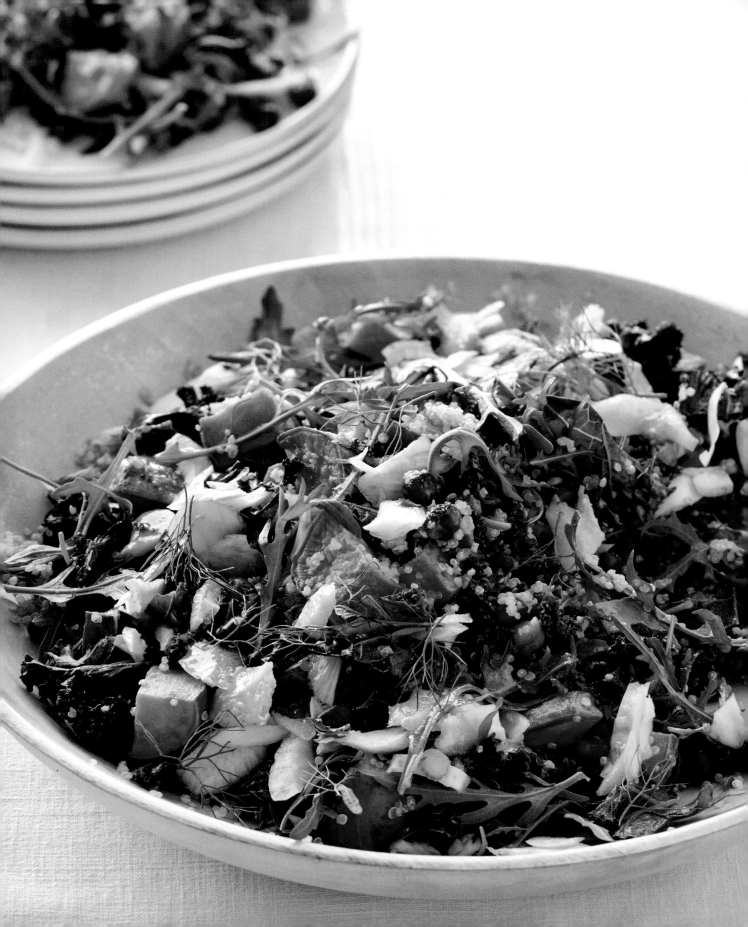

# SOUTHEAST ASIAN–INSPIRED NOODLE SALAD

**SERVES 4**

Tana loves noodle salads full of crunchy veg, nuts, and fresh herbs, with that unmistakable Asian-style dressing made of lime, fish sauce, and chiles, so there is often a big bowl made up in the fridge at home. I'm also a fan, as they are light yet filling and full of crunch and flavor. You could stir through some shredded poached chicken or sticks of mozzarella to add extra protein.

7 ounces brown rice vermicelli noodles
½ cup roasted unsalted peanuts, roughly chopped
3 carrots
1 medium cucumber, julienned
3½ ounces radishes, trimmed and sliced
2 spring onions, trimmed and finely chopped
½ bunch of cilantro, stems and leaves chopped
Small bunch of mint, leaves roughly torn

**FOR THE DRESSING**
Juice of 4 limes
2 teaspoons agave syrup
1 tablespoon fish sauce, or to taste
½ long red chile, seeded and finely chopped
   (optional)

| PER SERVING | |
| --- | --- |
| CALORIES | 386 |
| FAT (g) | 13.0 |
| SATURATED FAT (g) | 2.0 |
| CARBS (g) | 51.0 |
| SUGAR (g) | 10.0 |
| FIBER (g) | 6.0 |
| PROTEIN (g) | 14.0 |
| SODIUM (g) | 0.83 |

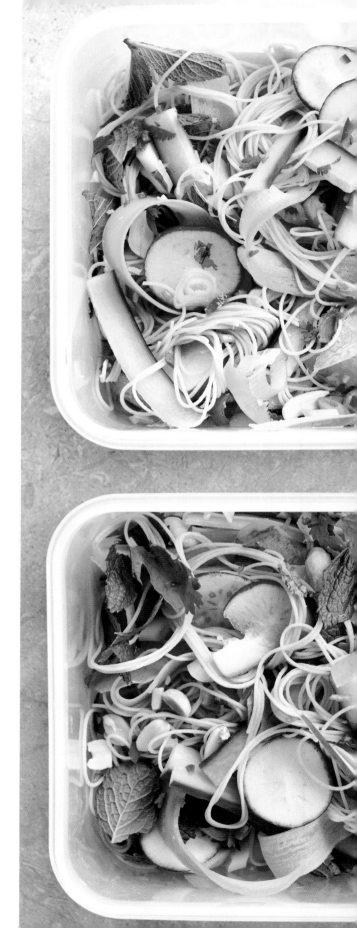

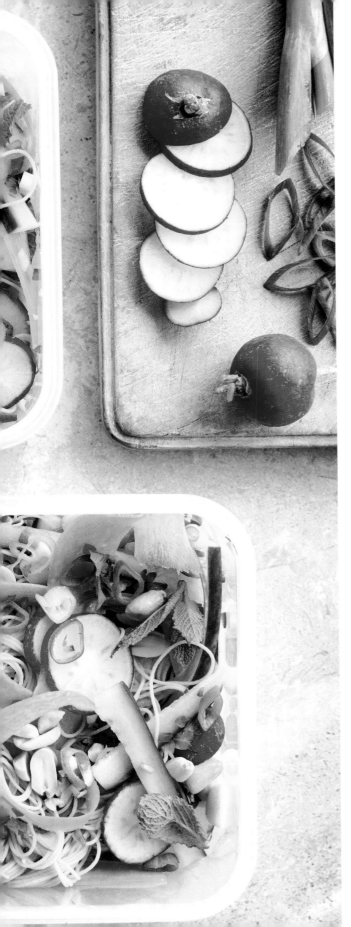

1. Soak the noodles according to their package instructions. Once softened, drain and run under cold water to cool.

2. Toast the peanuts in a dry skillet over medium heat until lightly golden.

3. Using a vegetable peeler, peel the carrots into ribbons and put them into the bowl with the cooled noodles. Add the cucumber, radishes, spring onions, cilantro, and mint to the bowl and toss really well to mix everything together.

4. For the dressing, mix together the lime juice, agave syrup, fish sauce, and chile, if using, then taste to check the balance (see below). Adjust the flavors as necessary.

5. Pour the dressing over the salad and add the toasted peanuts. Mix well, then serve or store covered in the fridge for up to 3 days.

**HOW TO BALANCE THE DRESSING**
For the dressing, you are aiming for a balance between sweet, salty, spicy, and sour, with no one ingredient being more pronounced than the other. For example, if you can taste lime juice more than any other ingredient, add a little more agave and/or fish sauce, and likewise with the other ingredients.

# SHRIMP WALDORF SALAD

**SERVES 4**

A classic Waldorf salad is a combination of crunchy apple, grapes, celery, and walnuts, which would be really good for you if it wasn't then coated with a thick layer of mayonnaise. Here I've added shrimp for extra protein and swapped the calorie-rich mayo for a much lighter Greek yogurt dressing, so you can have your Waldorf salad and eat it, too. The celery heart is the more tender inner stalks of the head that are often sold separately.

**FOR THE DRESSING**
½ cup Greek yogurt
1½ teaspoons Dijon mustard
1 teaspoon cider vinegar
Juice of ½ lemon, or to taste
Sea salt and freshly ground black pepper

**FOR THE SALAD**
½ cup chopped walnuts
1 small head romaine lettuce, finely shredded
7 ounces cooked, peeled shrimp, deveined
    if necessary
1 celery heart, chopped
1 tart apple, such as Granny Smith, cored and
    cut into ½-inch pieces
⅔ cup seedless green grapes, washed and halved

1. Start by making the dressing: Whisk together all the ingredients in a small bowl. Taste and adjust the seasoning as necessary, adding a little more lemon juice if needed.

2. Toast the walnuts in a dry skillet over medium heat for 2 to 3 minutes, until lightly browned.

3. Put the shredded lettuce leaves into a large bowl and add the shrimp, celery, apple, and grapes. Spoon in the dressing and toss to coat. Taste and adjust the seasoning as necessary before serving.

| PER SERVING | |
| --- | --- |
| CALORIES | 258 |
| FAT (g) | 16.0 |
| SATURATED FAT (g) | 3.0 |
| CARBS (g) | 10.0 |
| SUGAR (g) | 10.0 |
| FIBER (g) | 4.0 |
| PROTEIN (g) | 15.0 |
| SODIUM (g) | 1.14 |

**SALAD TO GO**
If you are taking this salad to work or on a picnic, dress it in the morning, but don't add the lettuce until you are ready to eat it.

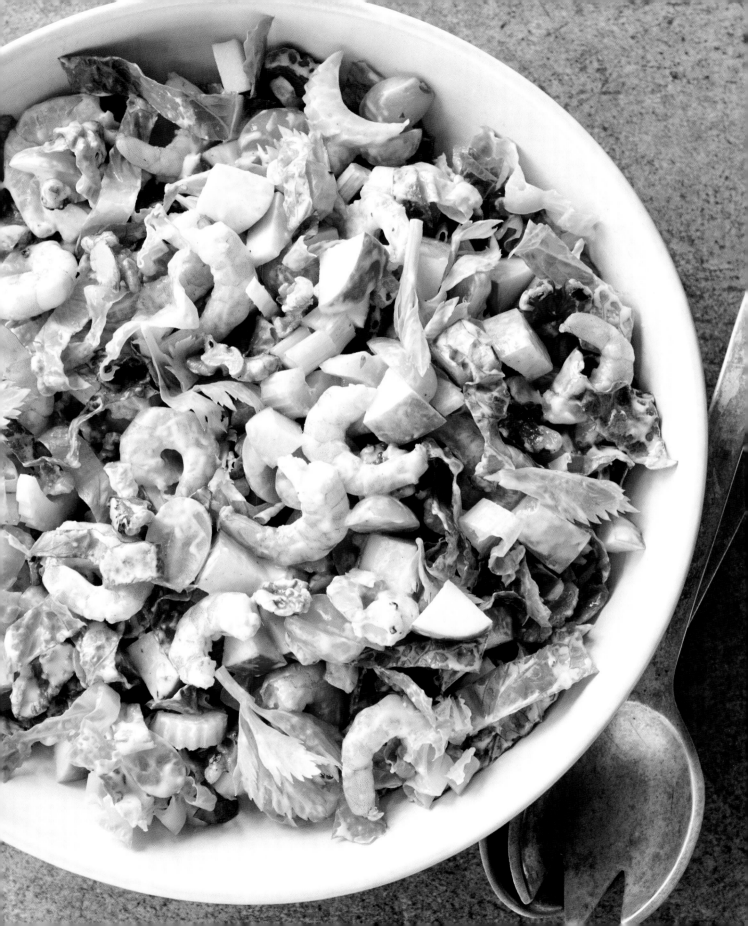

# TUNA AND AVOCADO TARTARE

**SERVES 4**

Tuna tartare looks really sophisticated and impressive, but you can pull it all together in a matter of minutes. Tuna is one of the oily fish, full of omega-3 fatty acids, that we are advised to eat at least once a week, and this makes a perfect light lunch with a green salad on the side. Make sure you get sushi-grade tuna that is as fresh as possible, and don't assemble the dish until just before you are ready to eat it; otherwise, the lime juice will "cook" the fish and turn it brown. Serve with an arugula salad and Pita Chips (page 266) to scoop up the tuna.

2 teaspoons tan or black sesame seeds
½ small bunch of chives, very finely chopped
1 tablespoon soy sauce
Juice of 1 lime
½ teaspoon toasted sesame oil
14 ounces tuna steak, cut into small cubes
Sea salt and freshly ground black pepper
1 large ripe avocado, peeled, pitted, and diced

**1.** Place a small skillet over low heat and toast the tan sesame seeds until golden and aromatic, then leave to cool. (There is no need to toast black sesame seeds.)

**2.** Put the chives, soy sauce, half of the lime juice, and the sesame oil into a mixing bowl. Add the tuna, season with a little salt and pepper, and toss to coat.

**3.** Put the avocado into another mixing bowl and gently fold in the remaining lime juice.

**4.** Divide the tuna among four plates, making a small mound of it in the center. Spoon the avocado on top, then sprinkle with the sesame seeds and serve immediately (see below).

| PER SERVING | |
| --- | --- |
| CALORIES | 224 |
| FAT (g) | 12.0 |
| SATURATED FAT (g) | 3.0 |
| CARBS (g) | 2.0 |
| SUGAR (g) | 1.0 |
| FIBER (g) | 3.0 |
| PROTEIN (g) | 27.0 |
| SODIUM (g) | 0.69 |

**HOW TO DRESS THIS UP**
To plate this as we do in the restaurant, rub the inside of a 2½- to 3-inch round pastry ring with a little extra sesame oil and place it in the center of a serving plate. Spoon in a quarter of the tuna tartare, add a quarter of the diced avocado on top, and sprinkle with sesame seeds, then gently and slowly remove the ring.

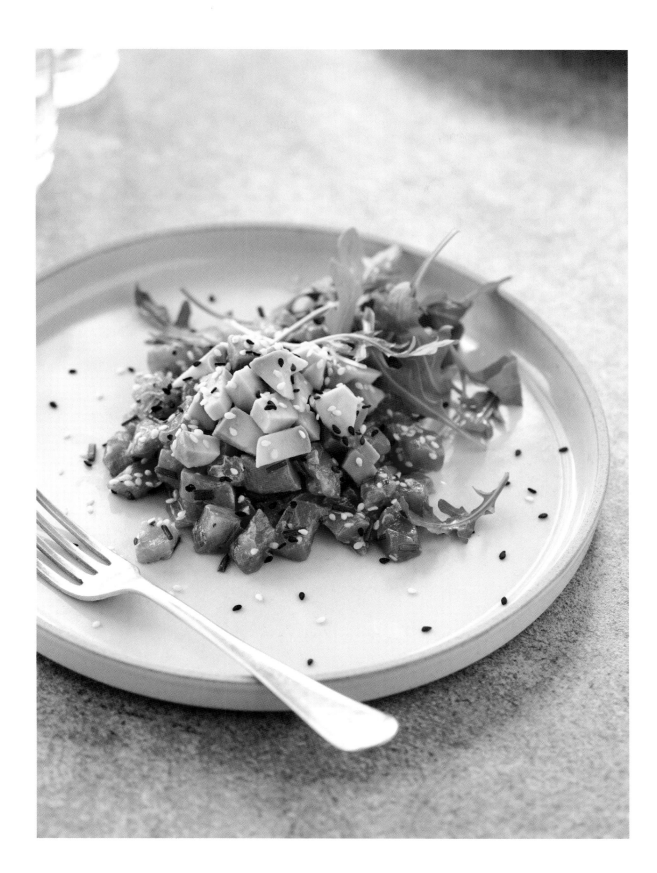

# HEALTHY VEGETABLE SAMOSAS

**SERVES 4 (MAKES 16 SAMOSAS)**

"Healthy" and "samosa" aren't two words I'd expect to see in the same sentence, but these are samosas with a difference . . . They are made with rice paper spring roll wrappers rather than the traditional fatty pastry, then baked in the oven rather than fried so they don't absorb all that oil during the cooking. They're stuffed full of vegetables, too, so as samosas go these really are as healthy as they can be. My kids love them, so we make up big batches for after-school snacks for them and their friends.

1 ½ teaspoons garam masala
1 ½ teaspoons ground cumin
1 ½ teaspoons ground coriander
1 ½ teaspoons black mustard seeds
1 tablespoon coconut oil, plus extra for brushing
1 onion, peeled and diced
Sea salt
1 garlic clove, peeled and finely chopped
1-inch piece of fresh ginger, peeled and grated
1 small cauliflower, cut into very small florets (about ½ inch)
1 carrot, cut into ½-inch cubes
⅔ cup frozen peas, defrosted
Sea salt and freshly ground black pepper
16 rice paper wrappers

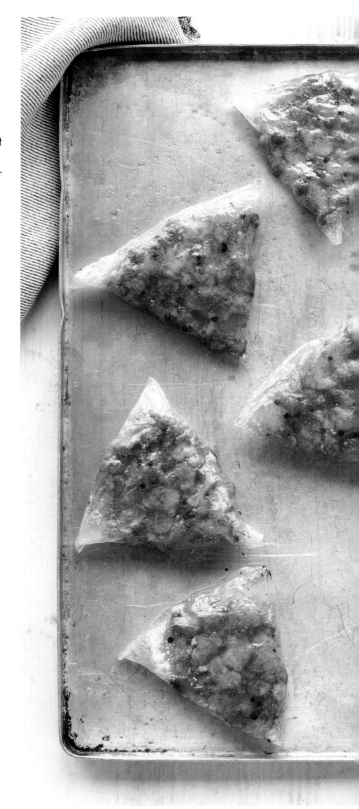

| PER SERVING | |
| --- | --- |
| CALORIES | 254 |
| FAT (g) | 5.0 |
| SATURATED FAT (g) | 3.0 |
| CARBS (g) | 42.0 |
| SUGAR (g) | 8.0 |
| FIBER (g) | 5.0 |
| PROTEIN (g) | 7.0 |
| SODIUM (g) | 1.14 |

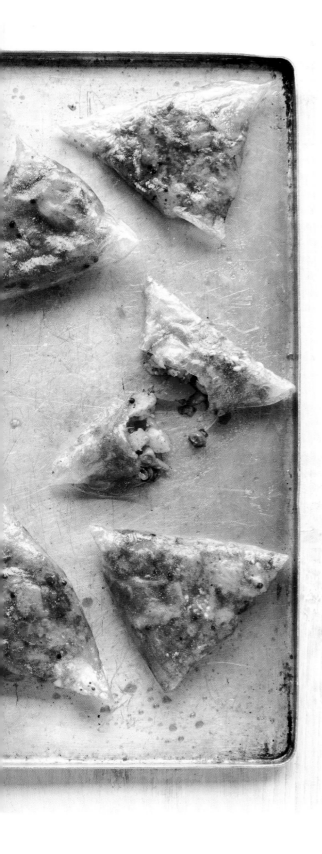

1. Preheat the oven to 400°F.

2. Place a large skillet over medium heat and add the spices. Toast for 30 seconds, or until aromatic, then add the coconut oil, diced onion, and a pinch of salt. Turn the heat down a little and sauté for 6 to 8 minutes, until softened.

3. Stir in the garlic and ginger and cook for an additional 2 minutes. Add the cauliflower and carrot and ½ cup of hot water. Turn the heat up a little and bring the water to a boil, stirring the vegetables until tender but still with a slight crunch (4 to 5 minutes).

4. Once the water has evaporated, add the peas and cook for an additional 2 to 3 minutes. Taste and adjust the seasoning as necessary, then remove from the heat and leave to cool.

5. Once ready to assemble the samosas, fill a shallow dish with warm water. Dip a rice paper wrapper into the water and leave until it becomes just pliable (don't let it get too waterlogged, as this will cause it to rip). Place the softened rice paper wrapper on a board and fold it in half to create a half-moon shape with the curved side to the right.

6. Place a heaping tablespoon of the mixture in the middle of the half-moon. Fold the bottom corner over the mixture two-thirds of the way up the curved side. Fold down the top corner to enclose the mixture, then fold over the edges to seal. The rice paper should still be wet enough to stick, but if it isn't, put a little water on your finger and run it along the edges before you fold and seal them. Repeat with the remaining mixture and rice paper wrappers.

7. Place the samosas on a baking sheet with the sealed edges facing downward and brush each of them with a little coconut oil. Put the sheet into the oven and bake for 10 minutes.

8. Remove from the oven, gently turn each of the samosas over, and brush the side facing up with a little more coconut oil. Return to the oven and cook for an additional 10 minutes.

9. Remove from the oven and eat while hot, or leave to cool and take on a picnic or in a packed lunch.

# SUPER
# SUPPERS
# AND
# SIDES

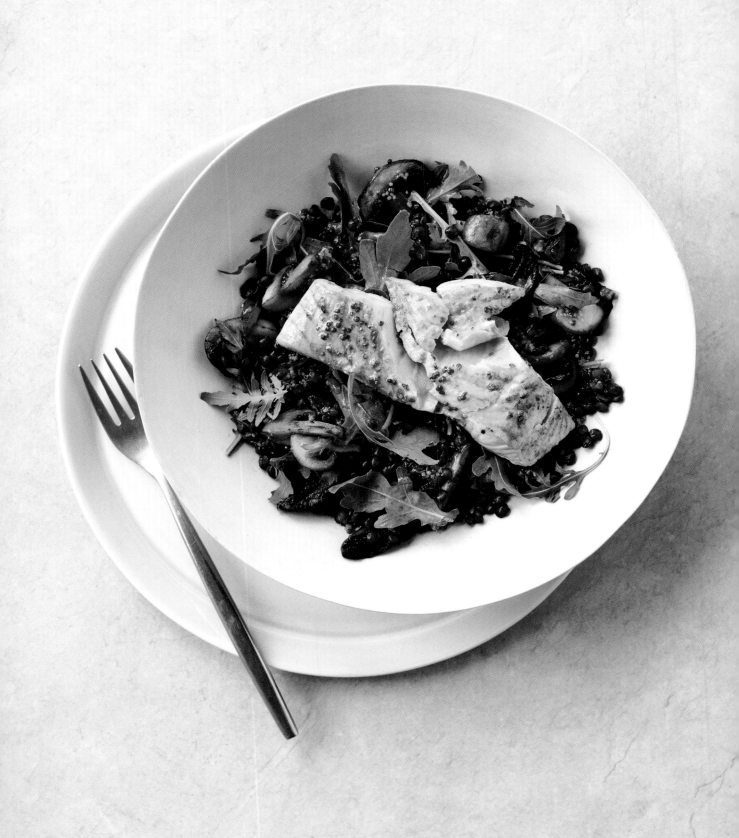

# GRILLED SALMON WITH GARLIC, MUSHROOM, AND LENTIL SALAD

**SERVES 4**

Winter salad may sound like a contradiction in terms, but this combination of lentils, mushrooms, and arugula is just that. It's a hearty, robust dish, perfect for autumnal and wintry days when regular salad ingredients are out of season. It's delicious on its own but is particularly good with grilled wild salmon, which also adds extra protein, healthy fats, and plenty of vitamins and minerals to your meal.

1 cup Puy lentils
1 bay leaf
2 thyme sprigs
3⅓ cups vegetable stock (or water)
1 tablespoon olive oil
7 ounces cremini mushrooms, cut into eighths
7 ounces portobello mushrooms, sliced
Sea salt
2 garlic cloves, peeled and finely chopped
4 (3½-ounce) wild salmon fillets
½ cup arugula leaves

**FOR THE DRESSING**
1 garlic clove, peeled and crushed
2 tablespoons white wine vinegar
1 teaspoon grainy mustard
1 teaspoon runny honey
1 tablespoon extra virgin olive oil
1 tablespoon water
Sea salt and freshly ground black pepper

1. Put the lentils into a large saucepan along with the bay leaf, thyme, and stock (or water). Bring to a boil over medium–high heat, then reduce to a simmer. Simmer for 15 to 20 minutes, until tender.

2. In the meantime, heat a large heavy-bottomed skillet over medium–high heat and add the olive oil. Once hot, add the mushrooms with a pinch of salt and cook for 6 to 8 minutes, stirring now and again, until soft and lightly caramelized on the edges.

3. Add the chopped garlic and continue to cook for 2 minutes, then remove the pan from the heat.

4. Once the lentils are tender, drain well and discard the herbs. Put the lentils into a large mixing bowl and add the mushrooms. Mix together gently to avoid breaking up the lentils too much.

5. To make the dressing, put all the ingredients into a clean jar with a pinch of salt and pepper. Close the lid of the jar and shake until the dressing comes together and emulsifies.

6. Preheat the broiler to high. Broil the salmon for 6 to 8 minutes, to your liking.

7. Pour half of the dressing over the warm lentils and toss gently to ensure everything is coated. Fold in the arugula, place the salmon on top, and pour over the remaining dressing. Serve immediately.

**HOW TO SAVE TIME**
To shorten the prep time, use canned lentils. For four people, you will need two (15-ounce) cans.

| PER SERVING | |
| --- | --- |
| CALORIES | 480 |
| FAT (g) | 20.0 |
| SATURATED FAT (g) | 3.0 |
| CARBS (g) | 29.0 |
| SUGAR (g) | 5.0 |
| FIBER (g) | 9.0 |
| PROTEIN (g) | 43.0 |
| SODIUM (g) | 0.78 |

# MISO COD EN PAPILLOTE

**SERVES 4**

Miso black cod, a Japanese favorite made popular around the world by the restaurant Nobu, is actually made with sable fish, which isn't cod at all. As it's difficult to get ahold of, I've come up with a way of using the same deep flavors with regular cod. This dish is fantastic for entertaining, as you can marinate the fish and make up the parcels in advance, then put them into the oven at the last minute. Let everyone open the parcels at the table so they get to smell the heady miso steam that comes out when they are opened. Serve with steamed rice and stir-fried vegetables.

¼ cup mirin
2 tablespoons white miso paste
1 tablespoon maple syrup
2 teaspoons soy sauce
4 cod fillets (approximately 4½ ounces each), skinned and pinbones removed
Olive oil, for drizzling
4 heads bok choy, leaves separated from the stem
1½-inch piece of fresh ginger, peeled and cut into matchsticks
4 spring onions, trimmed and thinly sliced

1. Mix together the mirin, miso paste, maple syrup, and soy sauce in a shallow dish. Add the fish fillets and turn to coat them in the marinade. Cover and leave to marinate in the fridge for at least 4 hours, or up to 2 days.

2. Preheat the oven to 350°F.

3. Drizzle four large pieces of foil or parchment paper with a little olive oil and place a pile of bok choy leaves in the middle of each square. Top with a layer of ginger and spring onions, then place the cod fillets on top, spooning over any remaining marinade.

4. Draw the edges of the foil or paper together, fold over to make a parcel, and seal tightly, leaving room for steam to circulate. Place the parcels on a baking sheet.

5. Bake in the oven for 10 to 12 minutes, until the fish is just cooked through.

6. Remove and leave to rest for a few minutes before putting each parcel onto a plate for your guests to open themselves.

| PER SERVING | |
| --- | --- |
| CALORIES | 171 |
| FAT (g) | 1.0 |
| SATURATED FAT (g) | 0.1 |
| CARBS (g) | 15.0 |
| SUGAR (g) | 10.0 |
| FIBER (g) | 3.0 |
| PROTEIN (g) | 24.0 |
| SODIUM (g) | 1.35 |

**GOOD TO KNOW**
As well as being delicious and nutritious, this dish is also low in fat, making it an excellent recipe for when you are watching your weight.

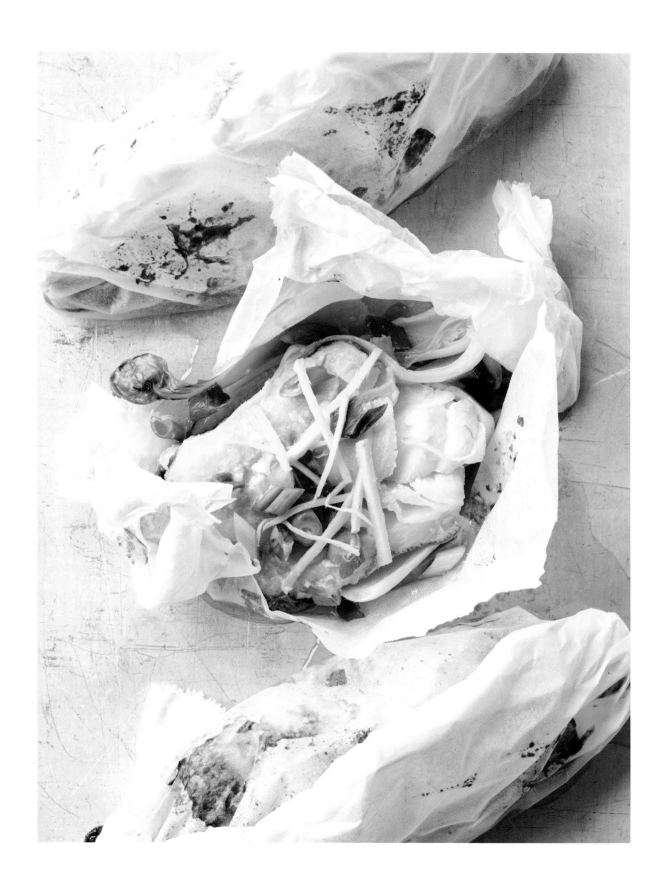

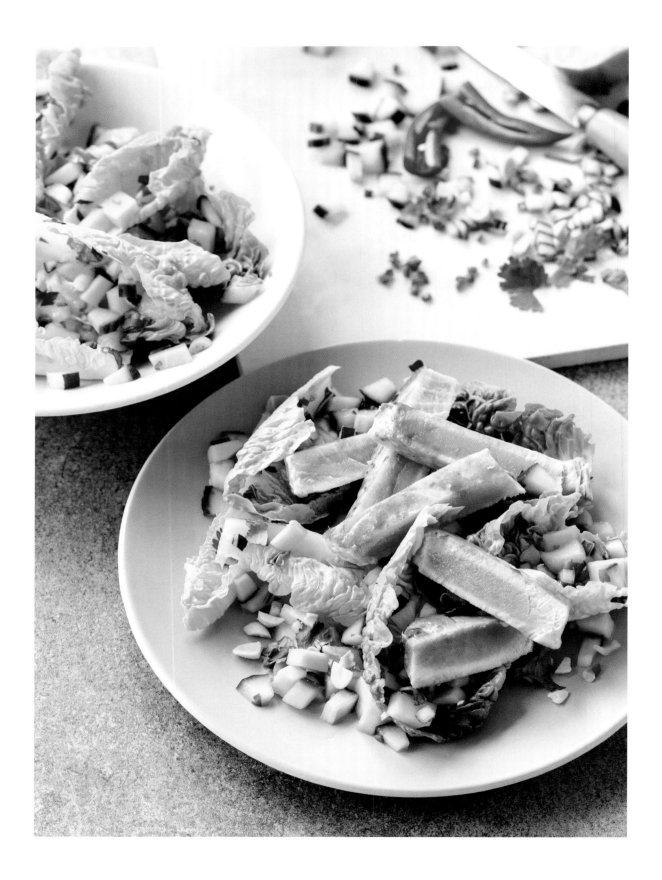

# TUNA STEAK WITH MANGO AND CUCUMBER SALSA

**SERVES 2**

Oily fish like fresh tuna are full of vital omega-3 fatty acids that are said to protect the heart as well as lower blood pressure and reduce fat buildup in the arteries. These essential fats are considered so good for you that the UK government recommends we eat at least one portion of oily fish every week. If you have fish-avoiding children, meaty tuna is a really good way to bring them around, especially when served with this delicious salsa—just leave out the chile if they don't like spice.

1 small mango, peeled and finely diced
1 small red onion, peeled and finely diced
½ cucumber, diced
½ small bunch of cilantro, roughly chopped
½ small bunch of basil, roughly chopped
2½ tablespoons unsalted peanuts, roughly chopped
1 red chile, seeded and finely chopped
2 teaspoons fish sauce
Juice of 2 limes
Olive oil, for drizzling
2 tuna steaks (approximately 6 ounces each)
Sea salt and freshly ground black pepper
2 Little Gem lettuce, leaves separated and washed

1. Mix the diced mango with the onion, cucumber, cilantro, basil, peanuts, and red chile. Pour in the fish sauce and lime juice and mix everything together. Taste and adjust the seasoning as necessary.

2. Drizzle a little olive oil over the tuna steaks and rub it into both sides of the fish. Season with salt and pepper.

3. Place a heavy-bottomed nonstick skillet over high heat. When hot, carefully put the fish into the pan and cook for 50 seconds on each side. Remove the fish from the pan and leave to rest for a couple of minutes.

4. Gently toss the Little Gem leaves through the salsa and pile up onto two plates. Slice the tuna steaks thickly, then place on top of the leaves and serve.

| PER SERVING | |
| --- | --- |
| CALORIES | 416 |
| FAT (g) | 13.0 |
| SATURATED FAT (g) | 2.0 |
| CARBS (g) | 18.0 |
| SUGAR (g) | 15.0 |
| FIBER (g) | 6.0 |
| PROTEIN (g) | 54.0 |
| SODIUM (g) | 1.36 |

# BEEF TENDERLOIN WITH LIMA BEAN AND FENNEL PURÉE

**SERVES 2**

Being healthy doesn't mean compromising on flavor. Take this knockout way of serving steak with a rich, velvety purée, intense oyster mushrooms, and crispy kale—it's as impressive as it is delicious. Serve it up for a special birthday or anniversary, or increase the quantities for a dinner party, and no one will even realize how healthy their food is as they tuck in.

1½ teaspoons canola oil, plus extra for cooking the steaks
2 large shallots, peeled and diced
2 fennel bulbs, trimmed and roughly chopped (½-inch pieces)
1 fresh bay leaf
⅔ cup 2% reduced-fat milk
1 cup chicken stock
1 (15-ounce) can lima beans, drained and rinsed

2½ ounces (about 1 cup) kale leaves
Olive oil, for drizzling
Sea salt
2 beef tenderloin steaks (approximately 5 ounces each)
Canola oil
Freshly ground black pepper
5 ounces oyster mushrooms, roughly torn into ½-inch strips
1 tablespoon roughly chopped parsley
Juice of ½ lemon

**CONTINUED ON PAGE 70**

| PER SERVING | |
| --- | --- |
| CALORIES | 488 |
| FAT (g) | 18.0 |
| SATURATED FAT (g) | 5.0 |
| CARBS (g) | 24.0 |
| SUGAR (g) | 10.0 |
| FIBER (g) | 16.0 |
| PROTEIN (g) | 50.0 |
| SODIUM (g) | 0.69 |

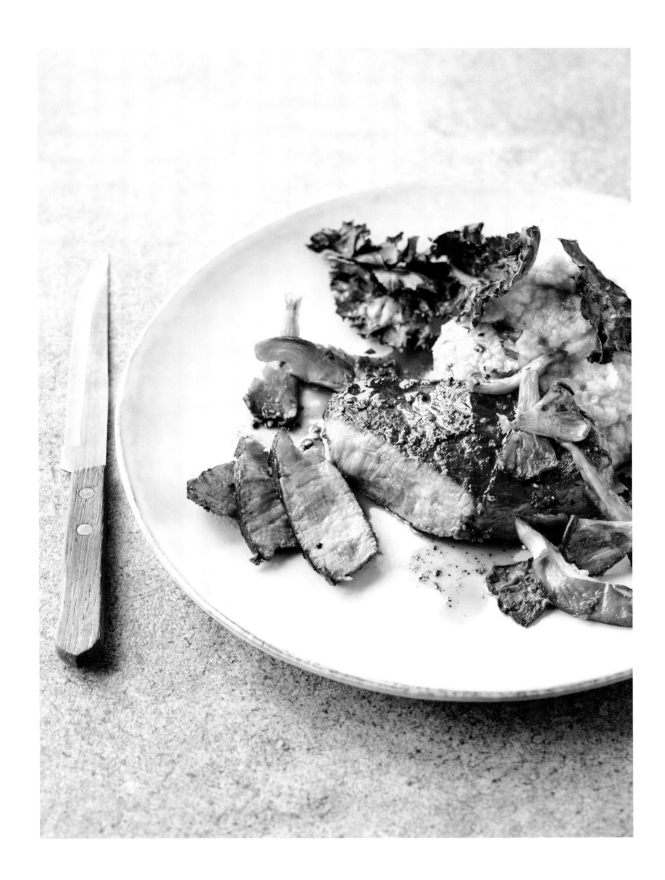

CONTINUED FROM PAGE 68

1. Preheat the oven to 325°F.

2. Place a saucepan over medium–high heat and add the canola oil. When hot, add the shallots, fennel, and bay leaf, lower the heat, and sweat for 8 minutes.

3. Pour in the milk and chicken stock and bring to a boil, then reduce to a simmer and cook for 10 minutes, or until the fennel is softened.

4. Add the lima beans and continue to cook for 10 minutes, or until everything is very soft.

5. Meanwhile, toss the kale leaves with a drizzle of olive oil and season with a small pinch of salt. Lay the leaves in a single layer on a baking sheet, place in the oven, and bake for 15 minutes, or until crisp. Remove and leave to cool.

6. Remove the bay leaf from the fennel and beans and pour the contents of the pan into a blender. Season with salt and blitz until smooth. If the purée isn't loose enough, add a little water and blend again.

7. Brush the steaks with a little canola oil and season all over with salt and pepper. Place a large skillet over high heat and, when smoking, carefully add the steaks to the pan and sear all over.

8. Transfer the steaks to a baking sheet and roast in the oven for 8 minutes for medium-rare. Remove the steaks from the oven, cover with aluminum foil, and leave to rest in a warm place for 10 minutes.

9. While the steaks are resting, add a little more canola oil to the same pan and place it over medium–high heat. When hot, add the mushrooms and cook, stirring occasionally, for 3 minutes, or until tender and lightly colored. Turn the heat off, season the mushrooms with a little salt and pepper, toss through the chopped parsley, and finish with a squeeze of lemon juice.

10. Serve the purée on two warmed plates and place the steaks on the side. Garnish with mushrooms and a handful of kale chips.

# BUTTERNUT SQUASH SPAGHETTI WITH SAGE AND WALNUT PESTO

**SERVES 4**

Making "spaghetti" out of sweet potatoes, zucchini, or squash is such a good way to increase your veg intake, and it looks brilliant, too. The sage and walnut pesto can be used with lots of other dishes, so make a double batch and keep it in the fridge for up to a week. It's great with chicken, Cornish game hens, or pork as well as roasted vegetables or stirred into a risotto.

**FOR THE SAGE AND WALNUT PESTO**
6 sage sprigs, leaves only
½ small bunch of flat-leaf parsley, leaves only
1 garlic clove, peeled and roughly chopped
½ cup walnut halves
Juice of ½ lemon
6 tablespoons extra virgin olive oil
Sea salt and freshly ground black pepper

**FOR THE SQUASH SPAGHETTI**
1 large butternut squash
Olive oil
1 garlic clove, peeled and finely chopped
Sea salt and freshly ground black pepper
Grated Parmesan cheese, to serve (optional)

1. Start by making the pesto: Put the sage, parsley, garlic, and walnuts into a small food processor and blitz until finely chopped.

2. Add the lemon juice and olive oil, season with salt and pepper, and process until emulsified (add a little warm water if the consistency is too thick). Taste and adjust the seasoning as necessary.

3. To make the butternut squash spaghetti, cut off the bulb at the bottom of the squash (save this for soup or the Roasted Butternut Squash, Farro, and Sumac Salad on page 45) and the stalk at the top. Peel the remaining part of the squash and use a spiralizer, julienne peeler, or mandoline to turn the butternut squash into spaghetti (see below).

4. Place a large skillet over medium heat and add a dash of olive oil. Add the chopped garlic and cook for 1 minute, then add the squash spaghetti. Toss over medium heat for 4 to 5 minutes, until tender but not soft, then remove from the heat and season with salt and pepper.

5. Stir in the pesto and transfer to warm serving bowls to serve. Sprinkle with grated Parmesan, if using.

**HOW TO MAKE VEGETABLE SPAGHETTI**
You can make vegetable spaghetti really easily with a gadget called a spiralizer. These are not expensive and are readily available online, but if you don't want to invest, use a julienne peeler or a mandoline with a julienne attachment. Just be careful of your fingers! For this recipe, try to buy a squash that has a long neck and smaller bottom (where the seeds are), as the neck part is what is used to make the spaghetti.

| PER SERVING | |
| --- | --- |
| CALORIES | 359 |
| FAT (g) | 31.0 |
| SATURATED FAT (g) | 4.0 |
| CARBS (g) | 13.0 |
| SUGAR (g) | 7.0 |
| FIBER (g) | 4.0 |
| PROTEIN (g) | 5.0 |
| SODIUM (g) | 0.02 |

# ZUCCHINI SPAGHETTI WITH MEATBALLS

**SERVES 4**

Zucchini noodles, or "zoodles," have been exploding in popularity. Zoodles with meatballs is filling and comforting, like a normal bowl of spaghetti, but it's particularly brilliant for all the family as you are upping your veg intake without compromising on flavor or texture. Zoodles are also great with pesto and other classic pasta sauces.

4 large zucchini, trimmed
Olive oil
Grated Parmesan cheese, to serve (optional)

**FOR THE MEATBALLS**
1 pound lean ground turkey
1 small onion, peeled and very finely chopped
2 garlic cloves, peeled and very finely chopped
2 teaspoons Worcestershire sauce
1 egg, beaten
Sea salt and freshly ground black pepper

**FOR THE TOMATO SAUCE**
Olive oil
1 onion, peeled and diced
2 garlic cloves, peeled and crushed
1 tablespoon tomato purée
1 (28-ounce) can chopped tomatoes
½ teaspoon dried oregano
½ teaspoon balsamic vinegar
Sea salt and freshly ground black pepper

| PER SERVING | |
| --- | --- |
| CALORIES | 291 |
| FAT (g) | 7.0 |
| SATURATED FAT (g) | 1.0 |
| CARBS (g) | 16.0 |
| SUGAR (g) | 14.0 |
| FIBER (g) | 5.0 |
| PROTEIN (g) | 39.0 |
| SODIUM (g) | 0.49 |

**FOR ACTIVE DAYS**
Serve the meatballs with whole-wheat pasta instead of zoodles if you are gearing up for a big day of exercise.

1. Using a spiralizer (see tip on page 71), julienne peeler, or mandoline, turn the 4 zucchini into spaghetti. Set aside until ready to cook.

2. Put the ground turkey into a mixing bowl with the chopped onion, garlic, Worcestershire sauce, beaten egg, and a good pinch of salt and pepper. Mix everything together until thoroughly combined.

3. With wet hands, roll the mixture into 20 meatballs and put them onto a plate. Cover with plastic wrap and chill in the fridge for 30 minutes.

4. Meanwhile, make the tomato sauce. Place a large skillet over medium heat and add a dash of olive oil. Once hot, add the onion and sauté for 5 to 6 minutes, until softened, then add the garlic and cook for another minute.

5. Stir in the tomato purée and continue to cook for 2 minutes, then add the chopped tomatoes, oregano, balsamic vinegar, and a good pinch of salt and pepper. Stir everything together and leave to simmer for 10 minutes, or until slightly thickened.

6. To cook the meatballs, place a skillet over medium heat and add a dash of oil. Once hot, brown the meatballs in batches, turning frequently so they color on all sides. Transfer to the pan with the tomato sauce to cook for an additional 10 minutes, or until cooked through, turning from time to time. (If the sauce becomes too thick, add about ¼ cup of water.)

7. Add an extra teaspoon of oil to the pan the meatballs were browned in and gently sauté the zucchini spaghetti over medium heat, tossing occasionally, for 3 to 5 minutes, until tender but not soft.

8. Divide the zucchini spaghetti among serving bowls and top with the meatballs. Sprinkle with Parmesan, if using.

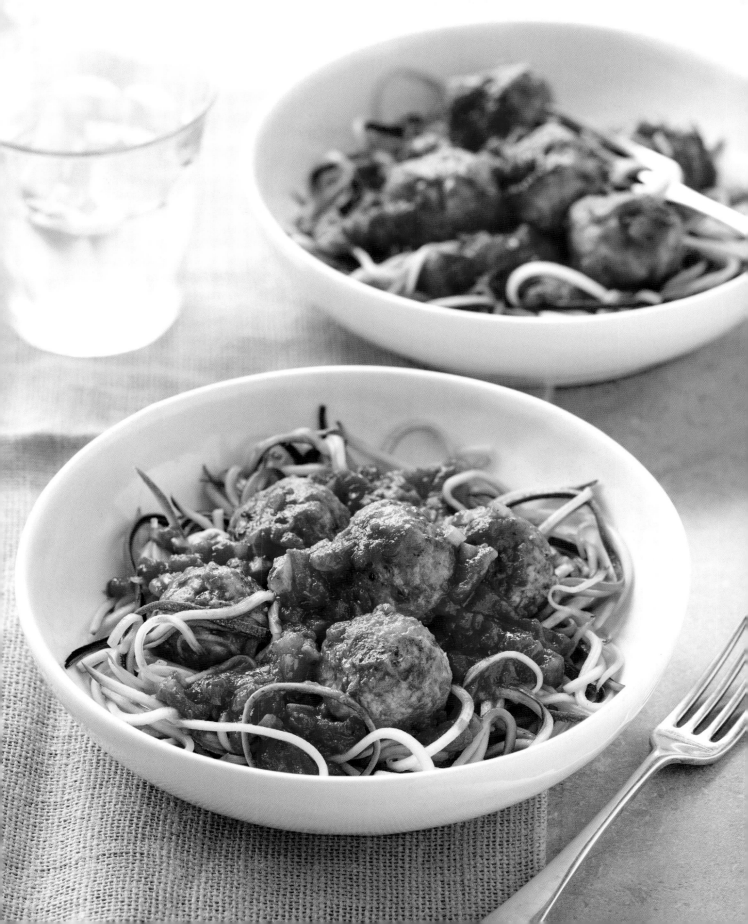

# LAMB STEAKS WITH CAULIFLOWER TABBOULEH

**SERVES 4**

Cauliflower is one of those vegetables that have a bit of a bad reputation. Most people avoid it unless it's smothered in cheese sauce and grilled. But evidence shows that we should all eat more cauliflower for its high levels of vitamin C and folic acid. By blitzing raw cauliflower in a food processer like this, it becomes like rice or couscous, with a crunchy texture that's perfect for a grain-free tabbouleh. (Of course, you can always add some cooked whole-wheat couscous or bulgur wheat to this salad if you are in training or building up to a race or match.) This is absolutely delicious with halloumi or chicken as well.

1 medium cauliflower, leaves removed
3 tablespoons extra virgin olive oil
8 ounces cherry tomatoes, quartered
1 small red onion, peeled and very finely diced
1 cucumber, finely diced
½ bunch of parsley
½ bunch of mint, leaves picked
Juice of 1 lemon
Sea salt and freshly ground black pepper
Canola oil
4 (4-ounce) lamb leg steaks, trimmed of excess fat
Lemon wedges, to serve

1. To prepare the cauliflower, either hold the stalk of the cauliflower and grate it on the large holes of a box grater, or break into florets and pulse briefly in a food processor until you get a rice-like consistency.

2. Put the cauliflower into a large serving bowl and drizzle with 1 tablespoon of the olive oil, then toss to coat.

3. Add the cherry tomatoes, red onion, and cucumber to the bowl and mix. Roll the bunch of parsley up tightly into a cigar shape and thinly slice the leaves until you reach the stems. Discard the stems, or save them for stock, and add the thinly sliced leaves to the bowl. Thinly slice the mint leaves and add them to the bowl.

4. Mix everything together well and squeeze over the juice of the lemon. Pour in the remaining olive oil and add a good pinch of salt and pepper. Mix well, taste, and add a little more olive oil or salt and pepper if needed.

5. Place a large skillet over high heat and add a dash of canola oil. When hot, add the lamb. Color for 2½ to 3 minutes on each side, until golden brown. Remove the meat from the pan and leave to rest.

6. Season the lamb with salt and pepper, then slice and serve with the tabbouleh and a wedge of lemon.

| PER SERVING | |
| --- | --- |
| CALORIES | 391 |
| FAT (g) | 20.0 |
| SATURATED FAT (g) | 5.0 |
| CARBS (g) | 11.0 |
| SUGAR (g) | 9.0 |
| FIBER (g) | 6.0 |
| PROTEIN (g) | 38.0 |
| SODIUM (g) | 0.26 |

**GOOD TO KNOW**
As a chef, I am used to peeling and seeding cucumbers, but given that the skin and seeds are packed with soluble fiber and other useful nutrients, it's worth keeping them intact here. Make sure you give them a good wash before eating, though.

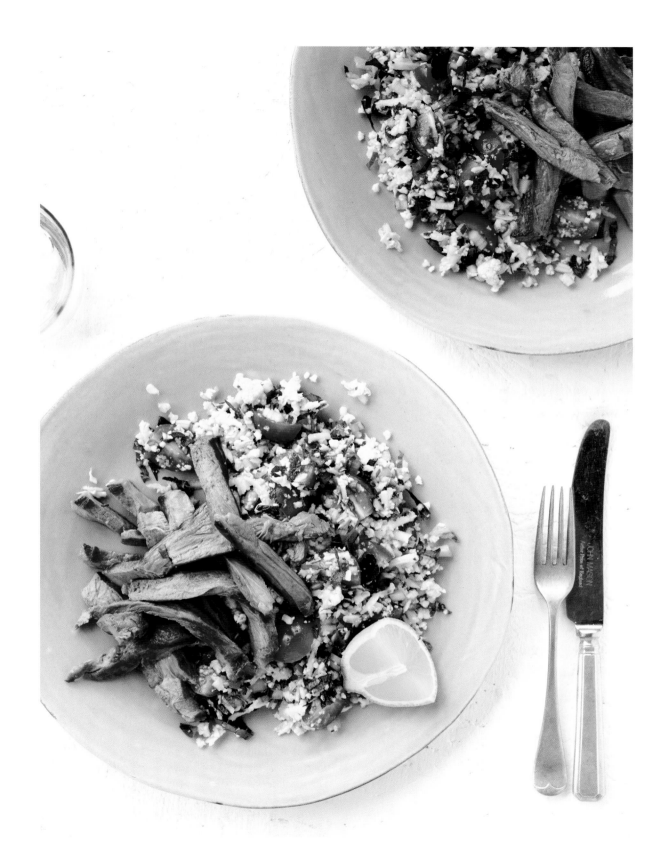

# SEA BASS CEVICHE WITH TOMATO, LEMON, AND CHILE

**SERVES 4**

Ceviche (raw fish marinated in lemon or lime juice) is a brilliant dish to eat when trying to be healthy— it is naturally low in fat but punchy in flavor, and because the fish isn't exposed to heat, it retains all the goodness that might be damaged during cooking. Make sure to use the freshest fish you can find—it makes all the difference to the finished dish. This is also good made with scallops, red snapper, or any other meaty white fish, and served with unsalted tortilla chips or toasted rye bread and a green salad.

14 ounces sea bass fillets, skin and pinbones removed, cut into bite-size chunks
¼ red onion, peeled and very thinly sliced
1 long red chile, seeded and finely chopped
Juice of 1½ lemons
4 medium ripe tomatoes, finely diced
½ small bunch of flat-leaf parsley, half the leaves picked, half finely chopped
Sea salt and freshly ground black pepper

1. Place the sea bass chunks, onion, chile, lemon juice, half the tomatoes, the finely chopped parsley, and a couple of pinches of salt and pepper in a large mixing bowl. Toss well to mix, then leave to stand for 10 minutes (or up to 30 minutes).

2. Once ready to serve, transfer the ceviche to a serving plate or shallow bowl and sprinkle over the remaining tomatoes and parsley leaves. Taste and adjust the seasoning as necessary, then serve immediately.

| PER SERVING | |
| --- | --- |
| CALORIES | 191 |
| FAT (g) | 10.0 |
| SATURATED FAT (g) | 2.0 |
| CARBS (g) | 4.0 |
| SUGAR (g) | 4.0 |
| FIBER (g) | 1.0 |
| PROTEIN (g) | 21.0 |
| SODIUM (g) | 0.19 |

**WHEN TO DRESS CEVICHE**
Don't dress the ceviche until you are almost ready to eat it; otherwise, the fish will "cook" in the acid of the lemon juice and lose its firm texture. Ideally the fish should be left to marinate for just 10 minutes, and definitely no more than 30.

# ZUCCHINI AND FENNEL CARPACCIO

**SERVES 4 AS A SIDE**

Finding new ways to include more vegetables, especially raw ones, in our diet can be challenging. Serving them in this way, very thinly sliced and "cooked" in a little lemon juice, is really simple, very refreshing, and deceptively impressive— especially when garnished with jewel-like pomegranate seeds, fresh mint, and black sesame seeds. It looks stunning! To make it a bit more substantial, crumble some feta or goat cheese over the top.

1 large fennel bulb
Zest and juice of ½ lemon
2 medium zucchini
Sea salt and freshly ground black pepper
2 tablespoons extra virgin olive oil
1 handful of mint leaves, thinly sliced
Seeds from ½ pomegranate
2 teaspoons black sesame seeds (optional)

**1**. Halve and thinly slice the fennel bulb, using either a mandoline or a very sharp knife. Put the wafer-thin slices into a bowl and squeeze over the lemon juice.

**2**. Using a vegetable peeler, peel thin strips from the zucchini and add them to the bowl with the fennel.

**3**. Season the fennel and zucchini generously with salt and pepper and drizzle with the olive oil. Toss to coat everything and leave to stand for 10 minutes.

**4**. After 10 minutes, toss through half the sliced mint leaves, taste, and adjust the seasoning as necessary, adding more lemon juice if needed, then arrange the salad on a serving plate. Scatter over the pomegranate seeds, lemon zest, and the remaining sliced mint leaves and finish with the black sesame seeds, if using.

| PER SERVING | |
| --- | --- |
| CALORIES | 106 |
| FAT (g) | 6.0 |
| SATURATED FAT (g) | 1.0 |
| CARBS (g) | 7.0 |
| SUGAR (g) | 6.0 |
| FIBER (g) | 6.0 |
| PROTEIN (g) | 3.0 |
| SODIUM (g) | 0.04 |

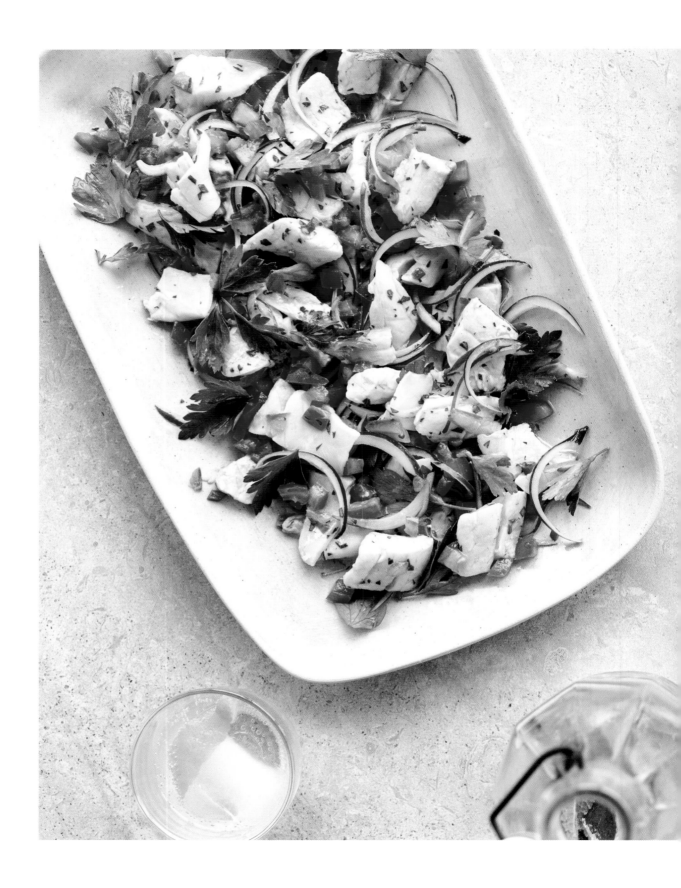

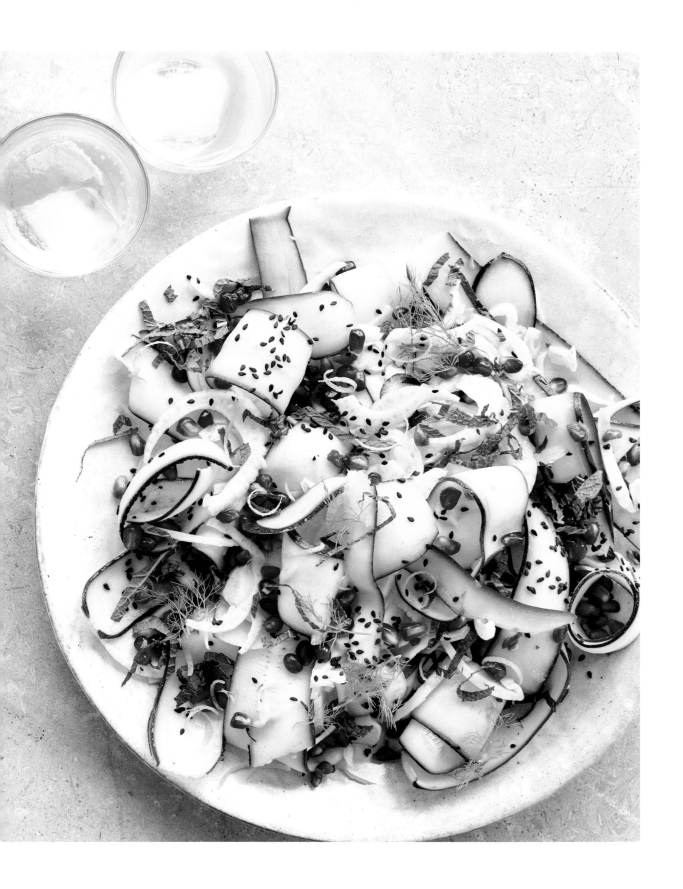

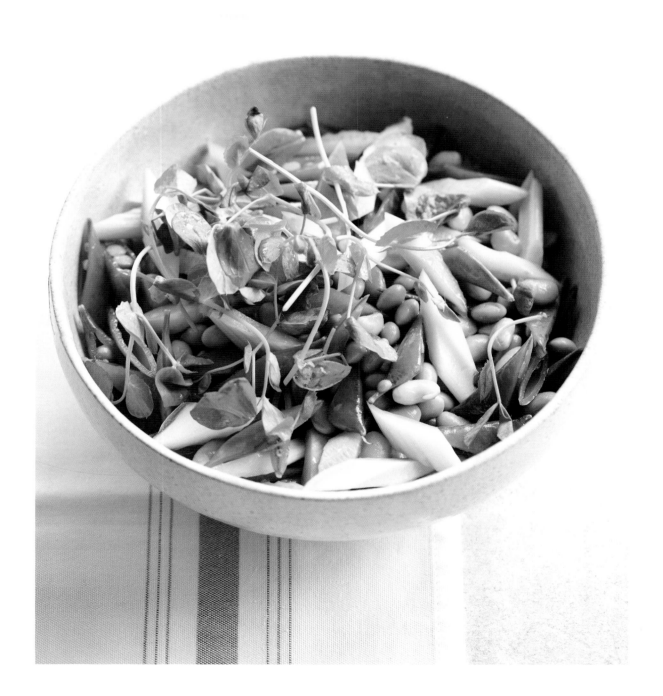

# EDAMAME, SUGAR SNAP PEA, AND CELERY SALAD

**SERVES 4 AS A SIDE**

This is a brilliantly vibrant green salad to add crunch to meat and fish dishes like the Miso Cod on page 64 or the Tuna Steak on page 67. You can buy edamame or fresh soybeans in their pods or shelled from some supermarkets these days, but if you can't find fresh edamame, buy the frozen beans—like peas they are frozen within hours of being picked so they are still full of nutrients.

12 ounces shelled edamame (fresh soybeans)
7 ounces sugar snap peas, topped and tailed
3 celery stalks, trimmed, any leaves reserved
Pea shoots, to garnish

**FOR THE DRESSING**
1 tablespoon rice vinegar
1 tablespoon soy sauce
1 garlic clove, crushed
2 tablespoons neutral oil, such as peanut

**1.** If the edamame need cooking, boil them in plenty of salted boiling water according to the package instructions. Drain and run under the cold tap to cool or place in a bowl of iced water to prevent further cooking. Once cooled, drain and pat dry.

**2.** Meanwhile, slice the sugar snap peas diagonally into thirds and put them into a bowl.

**3.** Halve each celery stalk lengthwise and slice on the diagonal into ½-inch-wide pieces. Put them into the bowl with the sugar snap peas and edamame.

**4.** Whisk together the ingredients for the dressing in a small bowl, then pour over the vegetables and toss well until everything is evenly coated. Serve immediately, garnished with the reserved celery leaves and pea shoots.

**HOW TO DEFROST FROZEN EDAMAME**
To defrost frozen edamame, put them in a microwavable bowl with a tablespoon of water, cover, and cook for 3 minutes, or as per package instructions, or blanch in a saucepan of boiling water for 3 minutes.

| PER SERVING | |
| --- | --- |
| CALORIES | 182 |
| FAT (g) | 10.0 |
| SATURATED FAT (g) | 2.0 |
| CARBS (g) | 8.0 |
| SUGAR (g) | 5.0 |
| FIBER (g) | 6.0 |
| PROTEIN (g) | 12.0 |
| SODIUM (g) | 0.64 |

# BAKED WHOLE TANDOORI-SPICED CAULIFLOWER

**SERVES 6 AS A SIDE**

Baking cauliflower whole in this way is so simple, but it looks really impressive. Make it the centerpiece of an Indian banquet and cut it open at the table as though you were slicing a cake. It's as tasty as it looks and yet it's incredibly easy to cook—just remember to allow a bit of time for the spiced yogurt marinade to really permeate the densely packed florets.

2 garlic cloves, peeled
¾-inch piece of fresh ginger, peeled
1 tablespoon tandoori masala spice mix
1 teaspoon cayenne pepper (optional)
Juice of ½ lemon
⅔ cup plain yogurt
Sea salt
1 medium cauliflower, leaves removed and base trimmed flat
Olive oil
Dried chile flakes, to serve (optional)

**1.** Using a fine grater such as a Microplane, grate the garlic and ginger into a large mixing bowl. Add the tandoori masala, cayenne (if using), and lemon juice and mix into a paste. Add the yogurt and stir thoroughly. Season well with salt.

**2.** Place the cauliflower, base side up, in the bowl. Using clean hands, spread the yogurt marinade all over the cauliflower, then leave it to marinate for at least 20 minutes, or up to 12 hours (cover the bowl and put it into the fridge if marinating for longer than 20 minutes).

**3.** When ready to cook, preheat the oven to 350°F.

**4.** Put the cauliflower, base side down, on a baking sheet rubbed with a little olive oil and pour over any extra marinade still in the bowl. Put the sheet into the oven and bake for 35 to 40 minutes, until golden and tender.

**5.** Put the cauliflower on a serving plate, sprinkle with chile flakes, if using, and slice it into wedges like a cake to serve.

| PER SERVING | |
|---|---|
| CALORIES | 66 |
| FAT (g) | 2.0 |
| SATURATED FAT (g) | 1.0 |
| CARBS (g) | 6.0 |
| SUGAR (g) | 5.0 |
| FIBER (g) | 2.0 |
| PROTEIN (g) | 4.0 |
| SODIUM (g) | 0.93 |

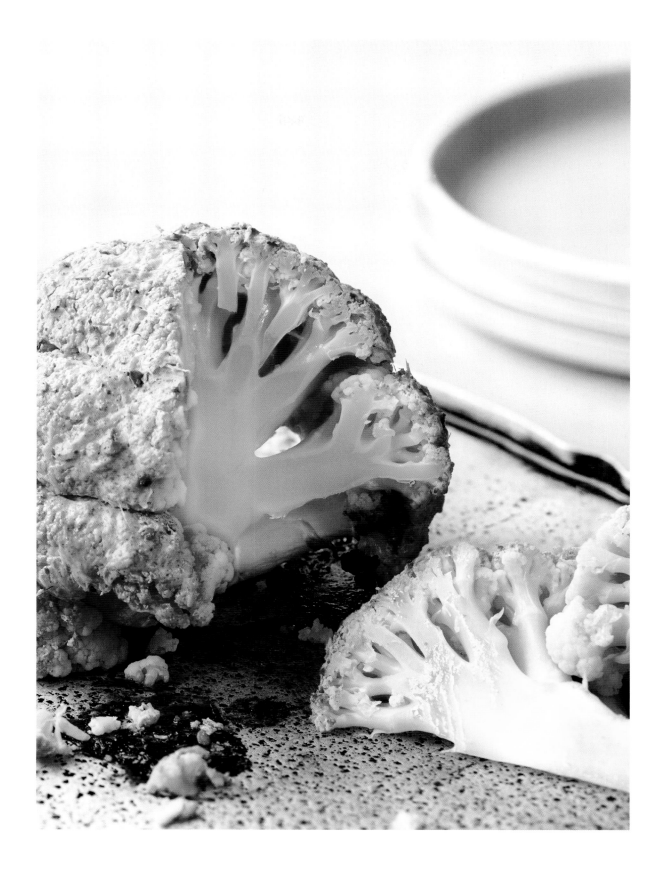

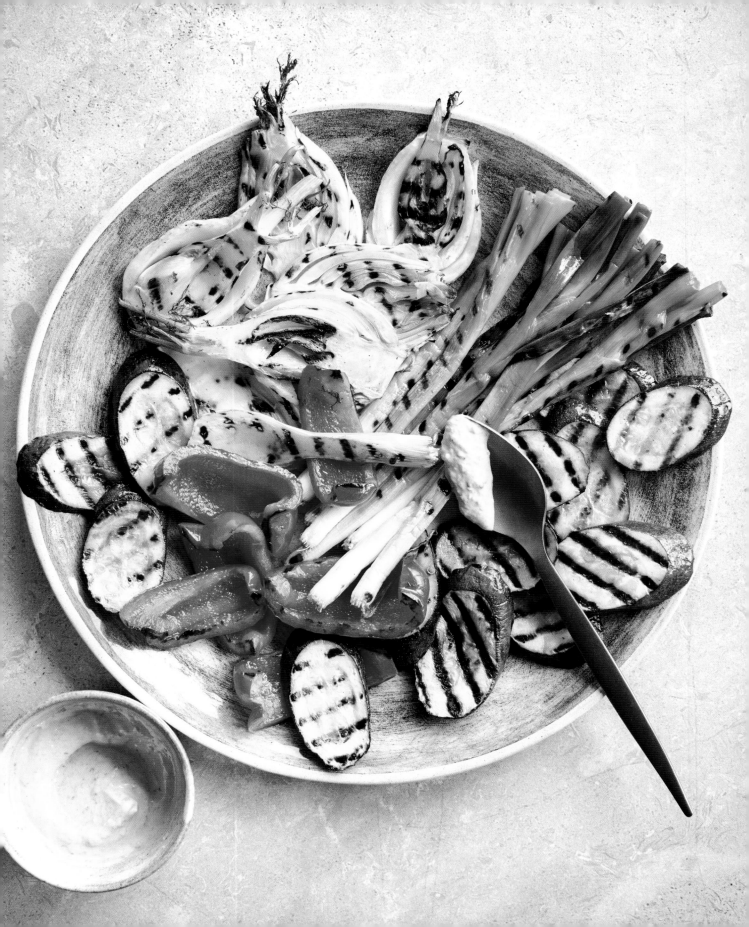

# CHARGRILLED VEGETABLES WITH BAGNA CÀUDA DRESSING

**SERVES 6 AS A STARTER OR SIDE**

Bagna càuda roughly translates as "hot bath" and refers to an intensely flavored hot dip popular in the Piedmont region of Italy. It is also great cold and makes a delicious dressing for raw or chargrilled vegetables and salads to accompany grilled chicken, fish, or lamb. This is a good dish to make ahead because the flavors really intensify over time.

**FOR THE BAGNA CÀUDA DRESSING**

1 (2-ounce) tin anchovies in extra virgin olive oil (oil reserved)
1 tablespoon capers, drained and rinsed
2 garlic cloves, peeled and roughly chopped
Zest and juice of ½ lemon
Freshly ground black pepper
¼ cup olive oil

**FOR THE VEGETABLES**

1 small fennel bulb, cut vertically into ½-inch-thick slices attached by the root
1 red pepper, seeded and cut into approximately 6 large pieces
2 zucchini, trimmed and cut diagonally into ½-inch-thick slices
8 spring onions, trimmed
Olive oil, for drizzling
Sea salt and freshly ground black pepper

1. To make the dressing, put the anchovies and their oil (apart from ½ tablespoon), the capers, garlic, and lemon zest into a small food processor and process until smooth.

2. Add the lemon juice with a pinch of pepper and mix together.

3. With the motor running, pour in the olive oil and about 3 tablespoons of cold water. Taste and adjust the seasoning if necessary.

4. Heat a grill pan over medium heat.

5. Put the vegetables into a bowl and drizzle with a little olive oil. Season with a pinch of salt and pepper and toss to make sure all the vegetables are coated.

6. When the grill pan is hot, grill the vegetables in batches until they are all tender and lightly charred. Transfer to a serving platter once cooked.

7. Drizzle the bagna càuda dressing over the vegetables or serve it in a separate bowl for dipping.

| PER SERVING | |
|---|---|
| CALORIES | 161 |
| FAT (g) | 14.0 |
| SATURATED FAT (g) | 2.0 |
| CARBS (g) | 3.0 |
| SUGAR (g) | 3.0 |
| FIBER (g) | 3.0 |
| PROTEIN (g) | 3.0 |
| SODIUM (g) | 0.85 |

# SHAVED ASPARAGUS AND HAZELNUT SALAD

**SERVES 4 AS A SIDE**

Shaving raw asparagus is such a good way to serve this favorite seasonal vegetable, and it makes a change from steaming or boiling it. Plus, it retains all its flavor, crunch, and goodness. The shavings make a great crisp salad that would be a lovely summer starter or accompaniment to grilled halloumi or creamy burrata.

½ cup blanched hazelnuts
3 tablespoons hazelnut or walnut oil (if unavailable, use extra virgin olive oil)
Zest and juice of ½ lemon
1 tablespoon white wine vinegar
Sea salt and freshly ground black pepper
1 pound thick asparagus spears

1. Toast the hazelnuts in a small, dry skillet over medium heat until golden. Remove and roughly chop, then set aside.

2. In a large mixing bowl, whisk together the hazelnut oil, lemon juice, vinegar, and a pinch of salt and pepper until combined. Taste and adjust the seasoning as needed.

3. Holding on to the woody end of the asparagus, shave the spears into long thin strips with a vegetable peeler or a very sharp knife. Put the shavings into the bowl with the dressing and gently toss to coat.

4. Place the dressed asparagus on a serving plate or in a bowl and scatter over the lemon zest and the chopped hazelnuts. Serve immediately.

| PER SERVING | |
| --- | --- |
| CALORIES | 196 |
| FAT (g) | 17.0 |
| SATURATED FAT (g) | 1.0 |
| CARBS (g) | 3.0 |
| SUGAR (g) | 3.0 |
| FIBER (g) | 4.0 |
| PROTEIN (g) | 6.0 |
| SODIUM (g) | 0.01 |

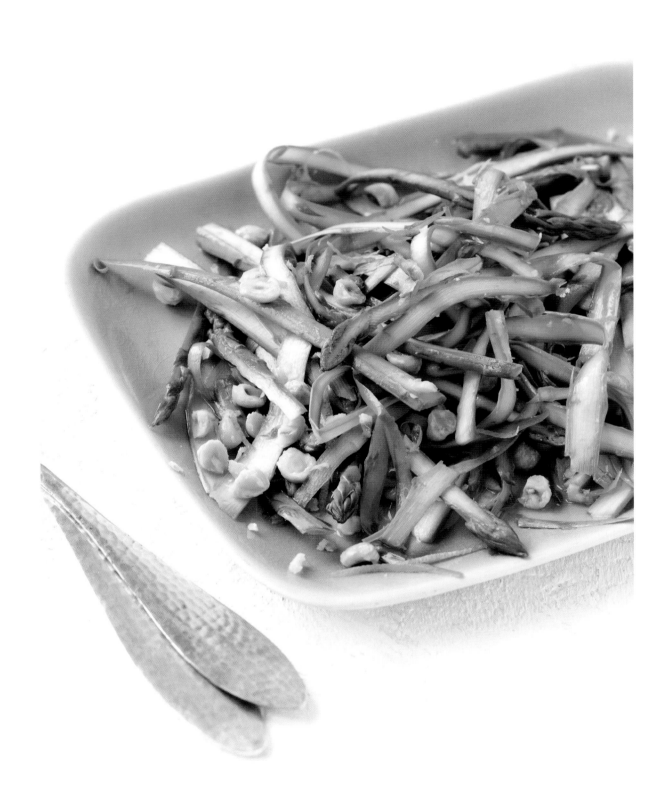

# HEALTHY SNACKS AND NOT-TOO-SWEET TREATS

# CUCUMBER AND MINT LEMONADE

**SERVES 4**

Homemade lemonade bears very little resemblance to the commercially produced stuff; it is less sweet and cloying and therefore much more refreshing on a hot summer's day. Adding the cucumber and mint makes it even more delicious and gives it an extra handful of vitamins and minerals, making it the perfect way to keep everyone hydrated.

½ cup lemon juice (from 2 to 3 lemons)
2 cucumbers, sliced
5 to 6 mint sprigs, leaves removed, plus extra
   to garnish
1 to 3 tablespoons agave syrup, to taste
Soda water
Lemon slices, to serve

**1.** Put the lemon juice, sliced cucumbers, and mint leaves into a blender and blitz until smooth, adding a little water if necessary. Once smooth, pour the liquid through a sieve or cheesecloth into a large pitcher, pressing the pulp with the back of a clean spoon to get as much liquid out as possible.

**2.** Taste the liquid and sweeten as necessary, stirring in the agave syrup a little at a time. Add a couple of handfuls of ice and top off with very cold soda water until it tastes just right (aim for roughly 1 part lemonade to 1 part water).

**3.** Serve chilled, with lots of ice, a slice of lemon, and a sprig of mint in each glass.

| PER SERVING | |
| --- | --- |
| CALORIES | 46 |
| FAT (g) | 1.0 |
| SATURATED FAT (g) | 0.0 |
| CARBS (g) | 6.0 |
| SUGAR (g) | 6.0 |
| FIBER (g) | 1.0 |
| PROTEIN (g) | 2.0 |
| SODIUM (g) | 0.02 |

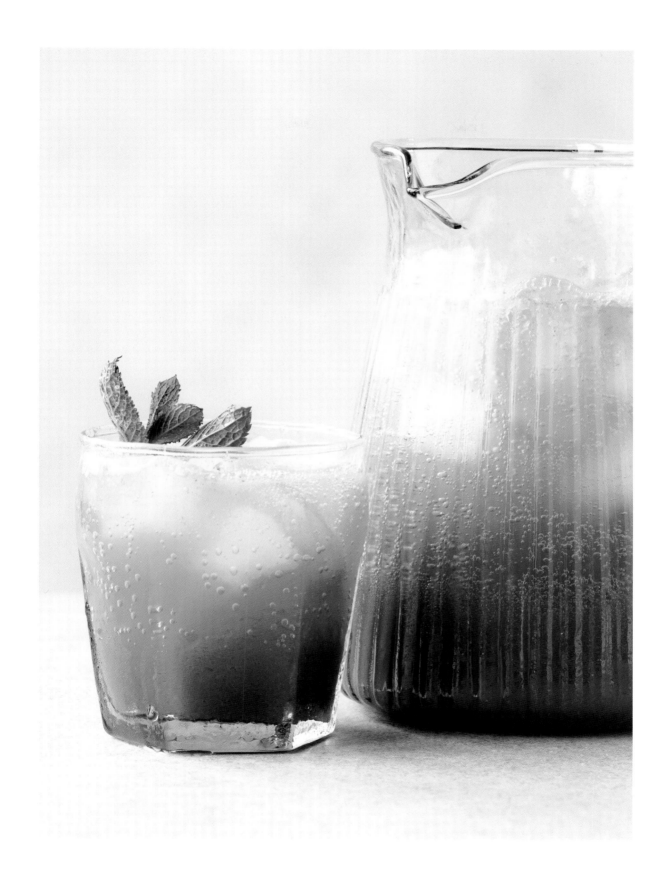

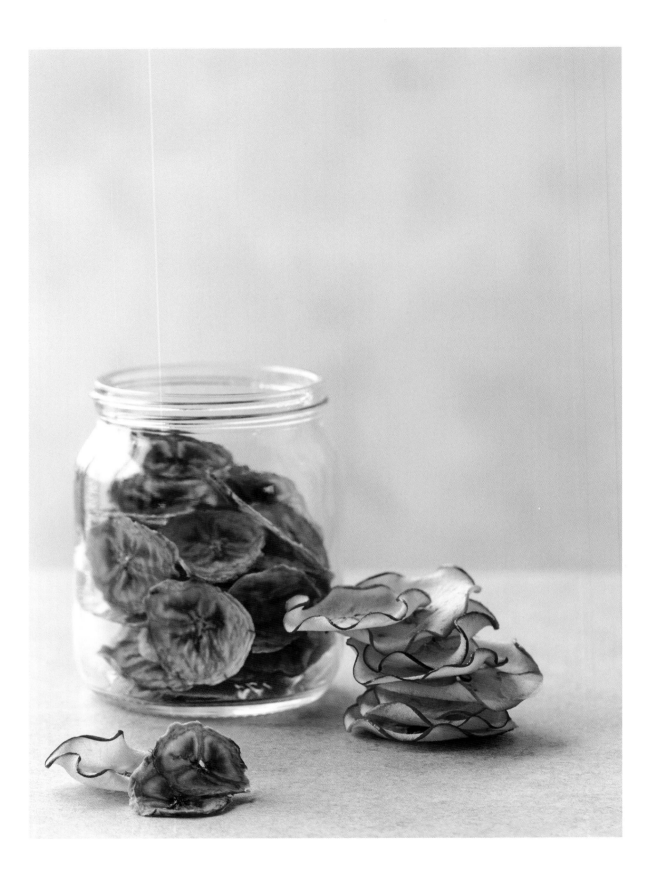

# BANANA AND APPLE CHIPS

**SERVES 4**

These healthy chips will provide both the sweetness and the crunch that we often crave when we're trying to eat more healthily and reduce our sugar intake. They make a great snack for kids, who end up eating lots of fruit without really realizing it. Great for adults, too, so make a big batch and keep them in an airtight container to last the week. These chips are also very low in fat, so add them to the list of guilt-free snacks starting on page 169 if you are watching your weight.

2 apples
2 bananas, peeled

**1.** Preheat the oven to 200°F.

**2.** Line 2 or 3 large baking sheets with waxed paper.

**3.** Slice the apples and bananas very thinly with a mandoline or sharp knife and lay the slices on the lined baking sheets in a single layer.

**4.** Put the sheets into the oven and bake for 1½ to 2 hours. The apples will be crisp before the bananas, so check them after 1½ hours. The bananas can take up to half an hour longer in the oven, depending on their thickness.

**5.** Leave the fruit crisps to cool on the sheet, then transfer to an airtight container and eat within 1 week.

**VARIATIONS**
This method also works really well for pineapple, pears, and star fruit, and you can try sprinkling the fruit with spices like cinnamon or cardamom for even more flavor.

| PER SERVING | |
| --- | --- |
| CALORIES | 70 |
| FAT (g) | 0.3 |
| SATURATED FAT (g) | 0.1 |
| CARBS (g) | 15.0 |
| SUGAR (g) | 14.0 |
| FIBER (g) | 1.0 |
| PROTEIN (g) | 1.0 |
| SODIUM (g) | 0.0 |

# SMOKY CANNELLINI BEAN HUMMUS

**SERVES 4**

Living in California for part of the year means my family and I have all developed a deep love of Mexican food. I find the smoky, hot flavors are creeping into familiar family dishes more and more, like in this cannellini bean hummus, which is seasoned with a very Mexican combination of chipotle chile paste, cumin, lime, and cilantro. It's now a favorite snack wherever we are.

Olive oil
1 small onion, peeled and diced
Sea salt
2 garlic cloves, peeled and roughly chopped
2 teaspoons cumin seeds
1 (15-ounce) can cannellini or other white beans, drained and rinsed
1 to 1½ teaspoons chipotle paste, to taste
Zest and juice of 1 lime
½ small bunch of cilantro, roughly chopped
Freshly ground black pepper

1. Heat a small skillet over medium heat and add a dash of oil. Once hot, sauté the diced onion with a pinch of salt for 5 to 6 minutes, until softened.

2. Add the garlic and cumin seeds and continue to cook for 1 to 2 minutes, until the garlic has softened and the cumin is fragrant. Remove the pan from the heat and transfer to the bowl of a food processor.

3. Add the beans, chipotle paste (starting with 1 teaspoon), a drizzle of olive oil (about ½ tablespoon), and the lime zest to the bowl and blitz until smooth. Taste and add a little more chipotle paste if you like it spicy.

4. Add half the lime juice and the chopped cilantro and blitz again until smooth with flecks of green. Taste and add a little more lime juice, salt, and pepper if necessary. Serve immediately, or store covered in the fridge for up to 3 days.

| PER SERVING | |
| --- | --- |
| CALORIES | 140 |
| FAT (g) | 3.5 |
| SATURATED FAT (g) | 0.0 |
| CARBS (g) | 20.0 |
| SUGAR (g) | 3.0 |
| FIBER (g) | 6.0 |
| PROTEIN (g) | 7.0 |
| SODIUM (g) | .43 |

**VARIATION**
Chipotle paste is available online and from many supermarkets. If you can't find it, replace it with 1 to 2 teaspoons of smoked paprika, stirring it in with the cumin.

# MINTED BABA GHANOUSH

**SERVES 4**

Eggplants are one of my favorite vegetables; they're so full of flavor, and making a creamy, smoky dip out of the flesh is a really good way of showcasing them. Serve this as a snack with crudités or Pita Chips (page 266) or as a side with grilled meats like sausages, lamb, and duck. The flavor of any dish made with eggplant improves over time, so this can easily be made two or three days ahead and will be more delicious for it.

2 medium eggplants
1 garlic clove, peeled and roughly chopped
1 tablespoon tahini
6 mint sprigs, leaves finely chopped
Juice of 1 to 2 lemons, to taste
Sea salt and freshly ground black pepper

**TO GARNISH**
Seeds from ½ pomegranate
2 mint sprigs, leaves thinly sliced

**1.** Turn on two burners. Place an eggplant directly over each burner, turning regularly until the flesh is soft and the skin is charred all over. Leave to cool.

**2.** Slice the eggplants in half and scoop out the flesh with a spoon. Put the flesh into a food processor and blend until as smooth as possible.

**3.** Add the garlic, tahini, mint leaves, and the juice of 1 lemon and season with salt and pepper. Blend again and taste to check the seasoning, adding more lemon juice if needed.

**4.** Serve the baba ghanoush in a bowl with the pomegranate seeds and sliced mint leaves sprinkled over the top.

---

**HOW TO CHAR EGGPLANT**
Lining your burners with aluminum foil before charring the eggplants will make cleaning up much quicker and easier. If you don't have a gas stove, roast the eggplants in an oven preheated to 400°F for 35 to 45 minutes, or turn them frequently under the broiler until really soft inside and blackened on the outside.

| PER SERVING | |
| --- | --- |
| CALORIES | 87 |
| FAT (g) | 3.0 |
| SATURATED FAT (g) | 1.0 |
| CARBS (g) | 8.0 |
| SUGAR (g) | 7.0 |
| FIBER (g) | 7.0 |
| PROTEIN (g) | 3.0 |
| SODIUM (g) | 0.01 |

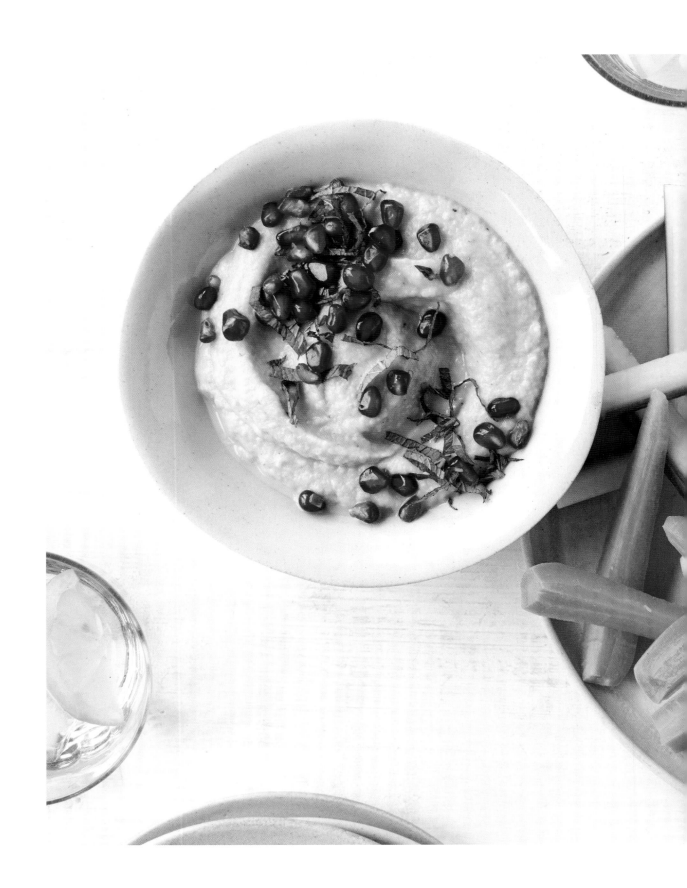

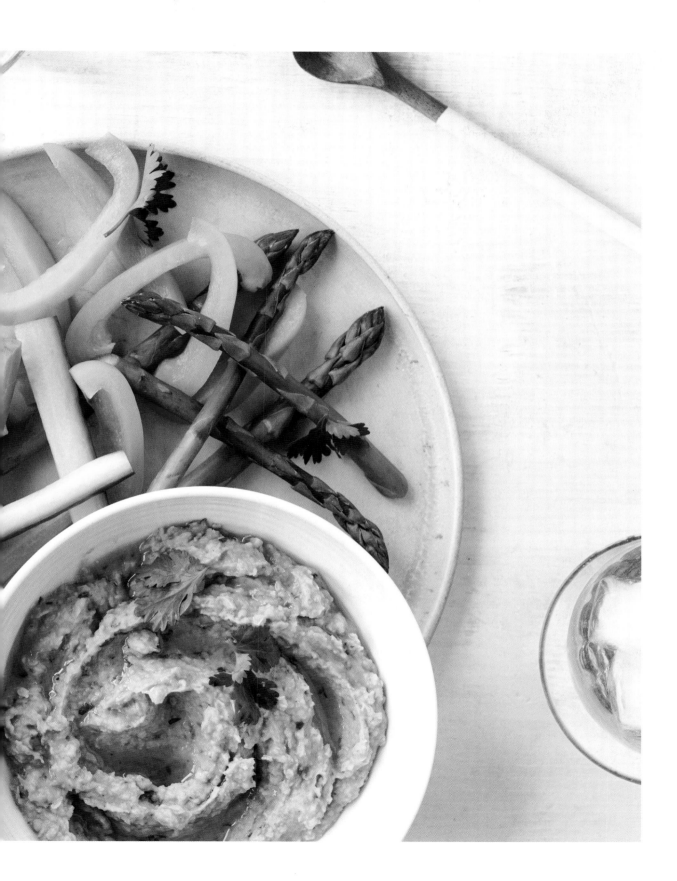

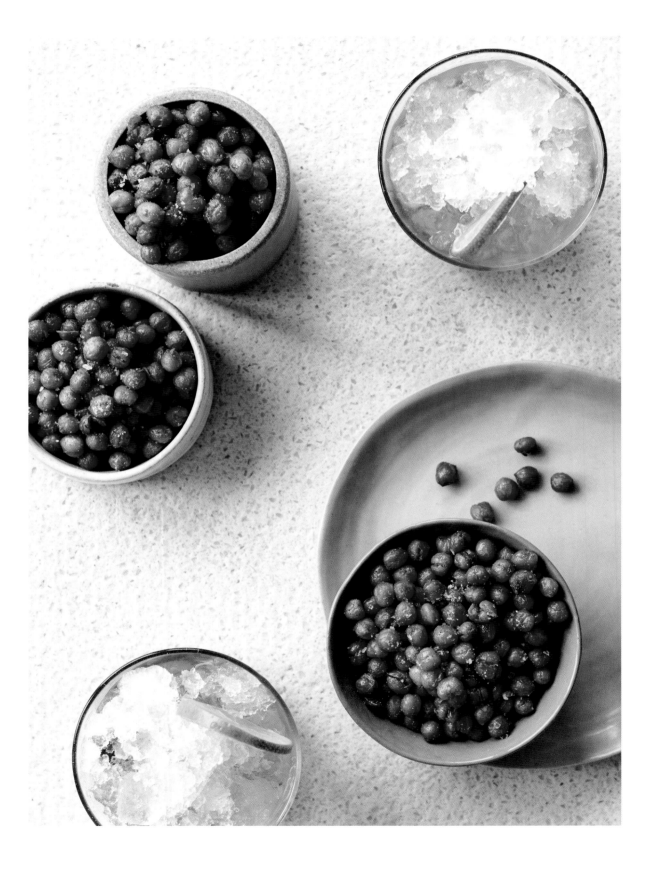

# CRUNCHY CHICKPEAS

**SERVES 4**

It's rare to find a satisfying savory snack to replace chips, but these chickpeas are just that—salty, spicy, and moreish, they really hit the spot with an evening drink or in front of a film. Double up the recipe for a crowd, as they are likely to disappear in seconds. Crunchy chickpeas are also a really healthy addition to salads and scattered on top of soups instead of croutons. Change the spices depending on your dish, or just season with salt and pepper.

2 (15-ounce) cans chickpeas, drained, rinsed, and dried very well
2 tablespoons olive oil
2 teaspoons ground cumin
1 teaspoon cayenne pepper (optional)
Sea salt and freshly ground black pepper

**1.** Preheat the oven to 350°F.

**2.** Make sure the chickpeas are completely dry, then spread them over two baking sheets. Drizzle with the oil and sprinkle over the cumin and cayenne pepper, if using, then season with salt and black pepper.

**3.** Put the sheets into the oven and roast for 15 to 20 minutes, until the chickpeas are completely crisp. Check them after 10 minutes and give the sheet a shake to move the chickpeas around.

**4.** Remove the sheets from the oven and allow the chickpeas to cool before serving. Store in an airtight container for up to 3 days.

**HOW TO MAKE CHICKPEAS CRISP UP**
The trick to getting the chickpeas really crisp is to make sure they are as dry as possible before you put them into the oven.

| PER SERVING | |
|---|---|
| CALORIES | 209 |
| FAT (g) | 9.0 |
| SATURATED FAT (g) | 1.0 |
| CARBS (g) | 19.0 |
| SUGAR (g) | 1.0 |
| FIBER (g) | 7.0 |
| PROTEIN (g) | 9.0 |
| SODIUM (g) | 0.01 |

# CHARGRILLED PEACHES WITH GRANOLA CRUMBLE

**SERVES 4**

This is a wonderfully summery dessert that is one of my daughter Tilly's favorites. It's a really simple, light dessert with a satisfying crunch and is the perfect way to end a summer lunch or barbecue. When peaches are out of season, you can replace them with ripe pears. The nutty granola crumble is also delicious sprinkled over yogurt or ice cream—it will keep up to ten days in an airtight container.

**FOR THE CRUMBLE**
⅓ cup rolled oats
1 tablespoon maple syrup
1 tablespoon coconut oil, or ½ tablespoon neutral oil, such as peanut
¼ cup almonds, roughly chopped
¼ cup pecans, roughly chopped
Pinch of sea salt
0% fat Greek yogurt, to serve (optional)

**FOR THE PEACHES**
4 ripe but firm peaches or nectarines, halved and pitted
Melted coconut oil or neutral oil, such as peanut, for brushing

1. Preheat the oven to 350°F.

2. To make the crumble, mix together the oats, maple syrup, and coconut oil (melted if necessary) until the oats are completely coated. Add the chopped nuts and a pinch of salt and mix again.

3. Pour the oats and nuts onto a baking sheet and bake for 7 to 10 minutes, until the oats are golden and crunchy.

4. Meanwhile, heat a grill pan over medium–high heat. Brush the cut sides of the peaches with a little oil and place on the hot grill pan, cut side down. Leave on the pan without disturbing for 3 minutes to allow the grill marks to develop.

5. Turn over and cook for another 2 minutes on the other side.

6. Serve the peaches warm, sprinkled with the nutty crumble. Serve with yogurt, if you like.

| PER SERVING | |
| --- | --- |
| CALORIES | 207 |
| FAT (g) | 13.0 |
| SATURATED FAT (g) | 4.0 |
| CARBS (g) | 17.0 |
| SUGAR (g) | 11.0 |
| FIBER (g) | 3.0 |
| PROTEIN (g) | 4.0 |
| SODIUM (g) | 0.13 |

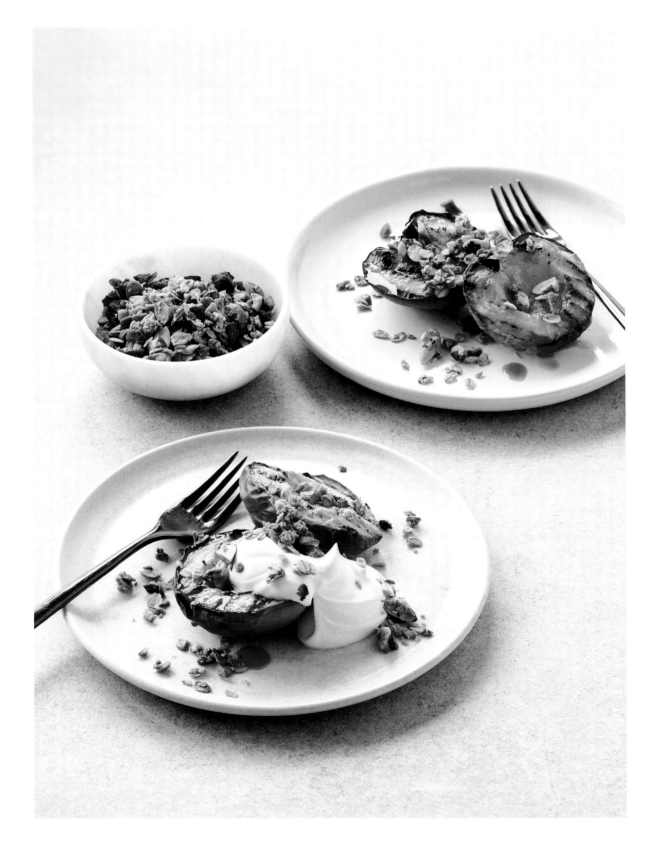

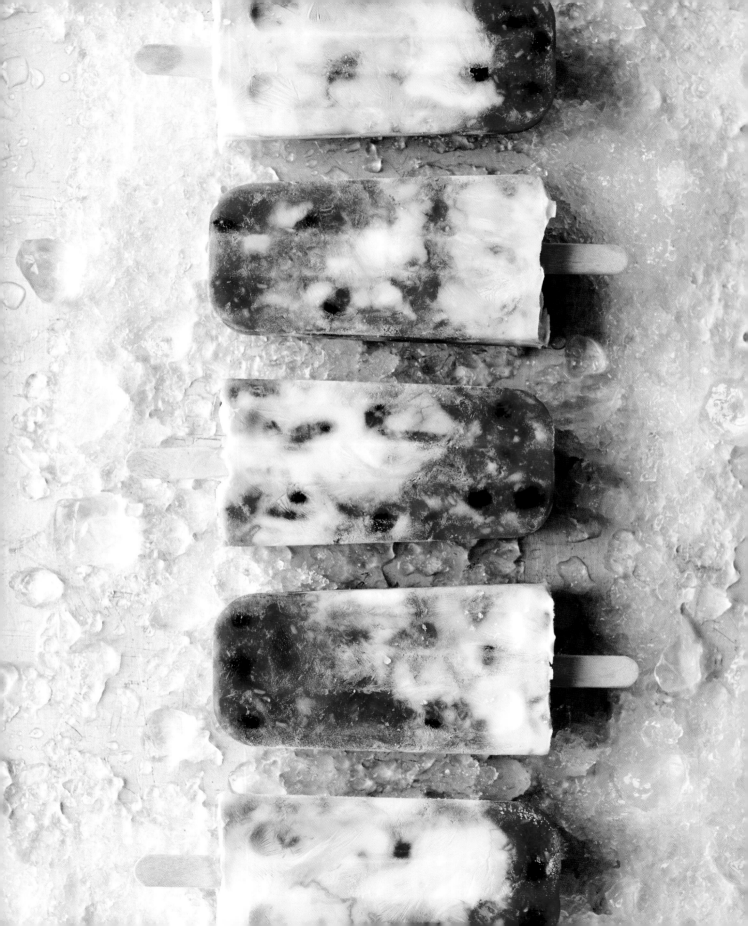

# YOGURT AND BERRY ICE POPS

**MAKES 6 ICE POPS**

This versatile recipe is a great way to get kids to eat more fruit in the summer and to avoid commercially made high-sugar ice pops and ice cream. Experiment with the flavor of the yogurt and swap the berries for diced banana, kiwi, mango, or melon, depending on what you have in your fruit bowl, but remember they take at least four hours to freeze solid.

3½ ounces fresh or frozen berries, such as strawberries, raspberries, or blackberries (defrosted if frozen), roughly chopped
1½ tablespoons runny honey
1¼ cups 0% fat plain Greek yogurt

1. Mash together the berries and half the honey with a fork until roughly puréed.

2. Put the yogurt into a bowl and mix in the remaining honey.

3. Spoon the mashed berries into the bottom of ice pop molds, then spoon the yogurt on top gently, mixing it together to create a ripple effect.

4. Put in the ice pop sticks and place in the freezer for at least 4 hours or overnight.

5. To serve, remove from the freezer and allow to warm slightly or hold under warm running water before trying to pull the ice pops out of the molds.

**GOOD TO KNOW**
These ice pops are low in fat and calories, so they can still be indulged in if you are trying to lose weight.

| PER SERVING | |
| --- | --- |
| CALORIES | 45 |
| FAT (g) | 0.0 |
| SATURATED FAT (g) | 0.0 |
| CARBS (g) | 7.0 |
| SUGAR (g) | 7.0 |
| FIBER (g) | 0.3 |
| PROTEIN (g) | 4.0 |
| SODIUM (g) | 0.14 |

# CHOCOLATE AND AVOCADO MOUSSE

**SERVES 8**

If you like a hit of sweet at the end of a meal, try this knockout chocolate mousse. It's made with avocado, which may sound strange, but it has a silky, creamy texture that really works with the chocolate. The result is a surprisingly decadent dessert that is so much better for you than the egg-based classic. And if you think people will turn their noses up when they hear about the avocado, don't tell them until they've finished it—they'll never guess!

2 large ripe avocados, peeled and pitted
3 to 4 tablespoons runny honey, to taste
1 teaspoon vanilla extract
½ cup raw cacao powder

**1.** Put the avocados into a food processor and process until smooth.

**2.** Add 3 tablespoons of the honey with the vanilla and cacao powder and process again until completely combined. Taste and add more honey if necessary.

**3.** Spoon the mousse into eight shot glasses or other small glasses and put them into the fridge for an hour before serving.

| PER SERVING | |
| --- | --- |
| CALORIES | 147 |
| FAT (g) | 10.0 |
| SATURATED FAT (g) | 2.0 |
| CARBS (g) | 10.0 |
| SUGAR (g) | 6.0 |
| FIBER (g) | 2.0 |
| PROTEIN (g) | 3.0 |
| SODIUM (g) | 0.02 |

**HOW TO MEASURE HONEY**
Because honey is so sticky, it can be difficult to measure it accurately—so much can be left behind on the spoon! If, however, you coat the measuring spoon with a thin layer of neutral oil like peanut, it will slip right off, ensuring that the right amount of honey makes it into your dish.

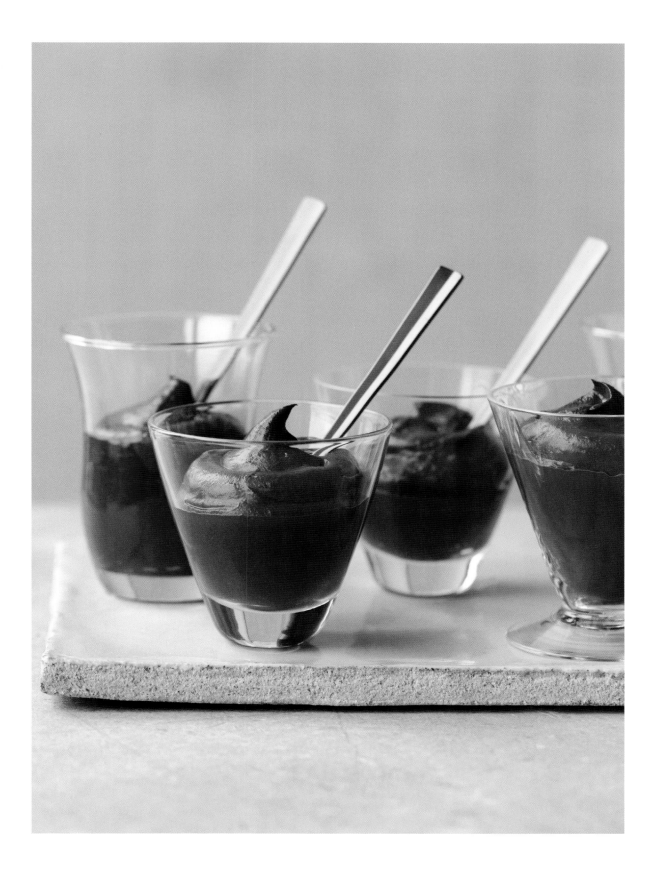

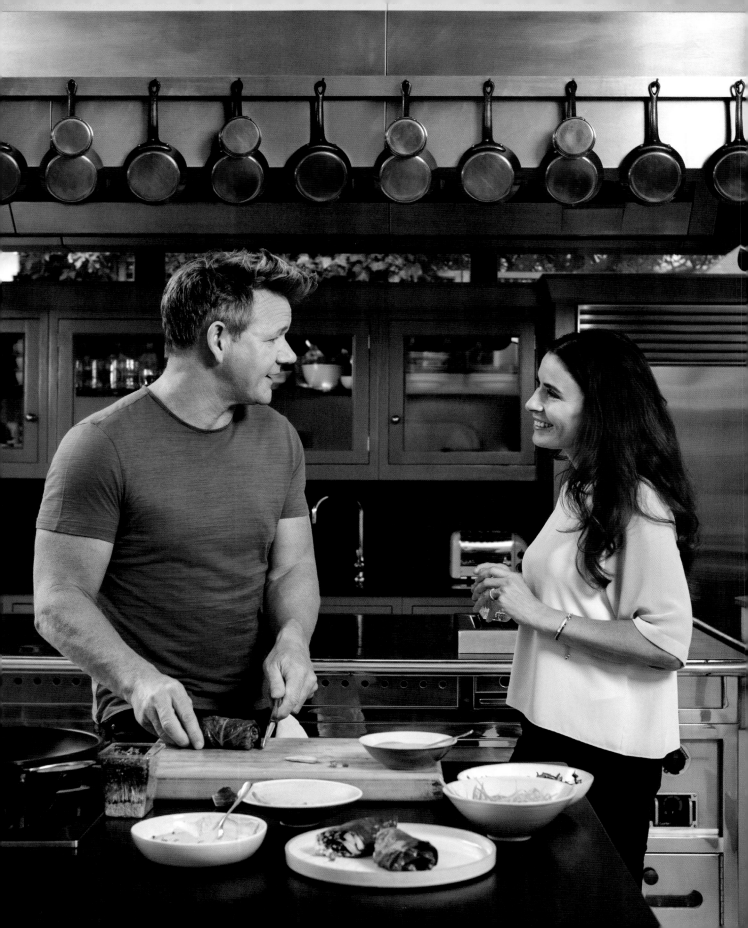

START-AS-YOU-MEAN-
TO-GO-ON BREAKFASTS

LIGHT LUNCHES TO
KEEP YOU ON TRACK

LEAN SUPPERS AND SIDES

GUILT-FREE TREATS

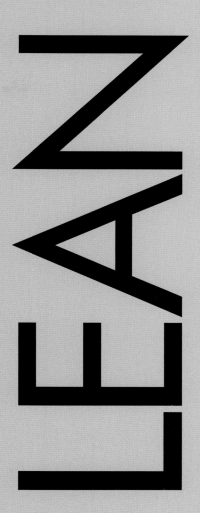

# THOUGH I HAVE LOST WEIGHT IN MY TIME, I HAVE NEVER REALLY BEEN ON A FORMAL DIET.

Maybe it's because I'm a chef, but I hate the idea of having to eat less or cutting out food groups or going hungry. Instead, I eat more carefully. I choose dishes and ways of cooking that are naturally low in fat and calories but big on flavor and satisfaction. I give favorite dishes a lean makeover and make sure I stock up on low-fat snacks. The trick for me is to not feel deprived and to enjoy the food I eat as much as I usually do. That, and to make sure I am getting plenty of exercise to burn up the food that I am consuming.

Essentially, the weight loss equation is really very simple. To lose weight, the energy generated by what you eat needs to be less than the amount of energy you are burning up through activity. If you are consuming more food than you are using, your body will lay down the excess as body fat. If you consume less than you need to, your body will use up this stored energy and you will lose weight.

Unfortunately, most adults consume more calories than they need, and while some people can get away with it, many of us are carrying around extra weight as a result. The simple solution is to eat less and start doing more exercise, but as that can sound a bit daunting, lots of people fail or don't even try. Personally, I like to think of it not as eating less but as eating better and getting more active, so that you can still eat many of the foods that you love.

Increasing activity levels will help you to lose weight faster, not simply because this burns up stored body fat but also because it increases your metabolism and, by replacing fat with muscle, you burn more calories while resting. But you don't have to start running ultramarathons—unless you want to, of course! Getting active can start with getting off the bus earlier than you need to, dancing around the kitchen, doing some gardening, or signing up for a charity run. The fitter you get, the easier exercise becomes, and the more weight you will lose.

I'm not saying it's easy. It involves willpower and determination and it won't happen overnight. The trick is to have manageable goals. When I needed to tackle my own weight gain, I didn't immediately sign up for an Ironman triathlon; I started running 5 km at the gym, then 10 km, and it went from there. When Tana was getting back into shape after our four children were born, she had a pair of jeans that she wanted to get back into. The thought of being able to fit into those jeans kept her going when it was tough.

This section is full of lean but satisfying dishes that we rely on at home to keep us on track. For me, the important thing is that they don't feel like diet food and I never feel like I'm depriving myself. There are sustaining salads, wraps, and soups; flavors from Japan, Vietnam, and North Africa; and even treats that are virtually guilt-free. It isn't easy, but this is a great place to start.

## ABOUT CALORIES

Personally, I have never counted calories. As a chef tasting lots of small mouthfuls all day, it would be impossible to add them all up! And I'm not necessarily suggesting that you count calories either, but it is a very useful way of judging food in terms of the all-important weight loss equation (i.e., the amount of energy consumed should be less than the amount used). Calories provide us with a clear numerical way of looking at food that can help to make this equation really straightforward.

Calories are basically a unit used to measure the amount of energy in food, and human beings need a certain number of calories per day to function. As a guide, an average man needs around 2,500 calories a day and an average woman needs around 2,000. As discussed, if you regularly consume more calories than this (and are only moderately active), over time you are likely to put on weight. If you are trying to lose weight, it is recommended that you reduce your daily allowance by 500 calories, to 2,000 calories per day if you are a man and 1,500 calories per day if you are a woman.

The calories in food come from macronutrients (carbohydrates, protein, fat), but each different macronutrient provides different amounts of calories per gram. Each gram of carbohydrate and protein provides 4 calories, while each gram of fat provides 9 calories. So you would have to eat more carbohydrates or protein to generate as many calories as fat. Or, to put it another way, cutting down on fat means you are consuming fewer calories more easily. The recipes in this section are generally lower in fat and sugar, to help you reduce your calorie intake by 500 calories a day, and they also include plenty of complex carbohydrates and lean proteins, to make you feel full and satiated and to keep you going in between meals.

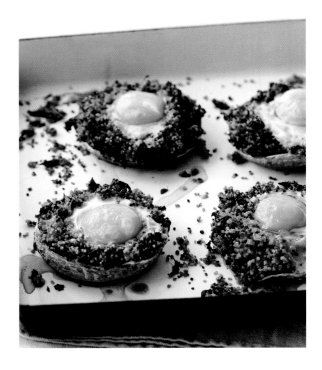

## A WORD ABOUT ALCOHOL

Recent studies have shown that drinking alcohol in moderation may actually be good for your health. Apparently up to three to five drinks a week may help prevent heart attacks and increase life expectancy, which, if it turns out to be true, could be great news for those of us who like a glass of wine now and again. The bad news is that alcohol contains 7 calories per gram, which is almost as much as fat, and that doesn't include the sugary mixers that often come with it. To put this into context, drinking five pints of lager a week is the equivalent of eating 221 doughnuts in a year! Plus, these are known as "empty calories" because they have no nutritional value whatsoever. On top of this, alcohol slows down the metabolism as the body prioritizes processing the booze rather than digesting food and burning energy.

So, if you are trying to lose weight, cutting back on alcohol is a really good way to keep your calorie intake down and your metabolism fired up. It's also much easier to stay on track if you don't drink; your resolve is immediately weakened by even one glass of wine or beer, and the food choices you make while drinking are often terrible. Then there's the hangover to contend with . . . If you really want to shift a few pounds, a dry period can help.

## EATING OUT

When I was working in the kitchen full-time, I obviously didn't get to eat in restaurants very often, but these days I have more evenings off and I love going out for meals with my family to celebrate special occasions or just to check out new chefs and dishes. The trouble is that I know only too well that chefs don't hold back when it comes to the fattening stuff like butter, cream, cheese, sugar, and chocolate. I don't want to feel deprived at home, let alone when I am out for dinner, so I set some rules that mean I can enjoy myself as much as everyone else. What follows is my advice for eating out when you are trying to stay slim.

Being starving hungry when you arrive at the table is a really bad idea, because you make terrible choices when you look at the menu and then tuck into the bread and butter, consuming half your allowed calories before the food even arrives! To avoid this, make sure you have a protein-rich lunch and a light afternoon snack to help you keep focused. If you don't want to eat anything beforehand, a clever trick is to look at the menu online, preferably when you aren't hungry, pick out the healthiest option, and don't even look at the menu when you get there.

I've already covered alcohol, but just say no to a sugary aperitif or cocktail before you eat and restrict yourself to one glass of excellent wine or a favorite beer to be enjoyed with the food. Getting tipsy on an empty stomach will definitely lead to bad choices, and more alcohol will add a lot of empty calories to an already indulgent meal. Say no to bread, too. Yes, it's really delicious, but as I have already said, you can consume lots of calories before your food has even arrived, and why pay to fill yourself up on something you can toast at home? You're there for the chef's expertise, so save your calories.

When we eat out as a family, everyone always wants three courses, so Tana and I share a starter and dessert, which keeps our overall intake down. If you aren't very good at sharing, choose a starter or a dessert rather than having both, or choose a second starter for your main course. If you can't resist something sweet at the end of a meal, order a cup of peppermint tea with a little honey stirred in, or have a square of dark chocolate on the way home. But if things go wrong and you just can't resist that chocolate mousse, go for an extra-long run the next day as penance!

# START-AS-YOU-MEAN-TO-GO-ON BREAKFASTS

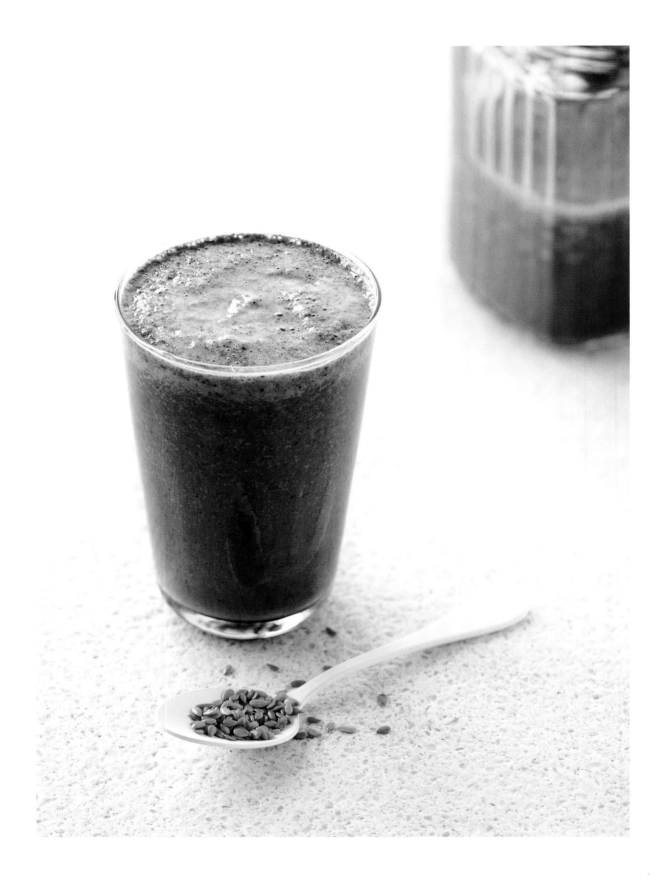

# BERRY AND OAT SMOOTHIE
**SERVES 1**

Adding oats and flaxseeds to a fruit smoothie will not only help you feel fuller longer but will also slow down the rate at which the natural sugars from the fruit hit your system, helping to avoid peaks and lows in blood sugar levels for the rest of the day. You can also add other fruits such as strawberries, raspberries, pear, banana, or mango, depending on what you have in the fruit bowl.

⅓ cup rolled oats
⅔ cup 2% reduced-fat milk
2 teaspoons honey
½ cup blueberries
½ cup blackberries
2 teaspoons ground flaxseeds

**1**. Put the oats into a blender and pour over the milk. Leave to sit for 5 minutes.

**2**. Add the honey, blueberries, blackberries, and ground flaxseeds and blitz until smooth.

**GOOD TO KNOW**
This would be a good pre-race or workout smoothie, too.

| PER SERVING | |
| --- | --- |
| CALORIES | 297 |
| FAT (g) | 8.0 |
| SATURATED FAT (g) | 2.0 |
| CARBS (g) | 41.0 |
| SUGAR (g) | 24.0 |
| FIBER (g) | 9.0 |
| PROTEIN (g) | 11.0 |
| SODIUM (g) | 0.18 |

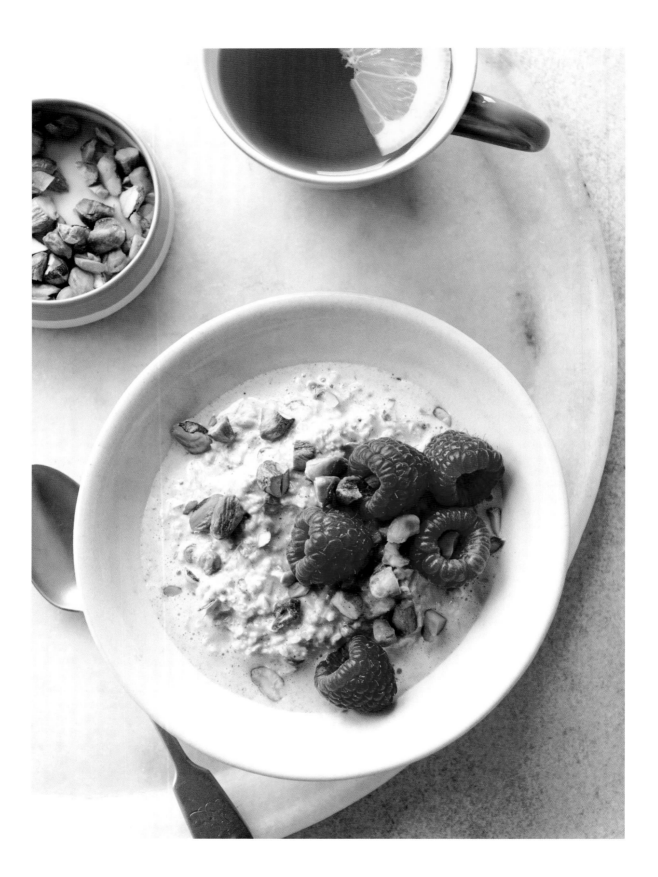

# RASPBERRY AND HONEY OVERNIGHT OATS

**SERVES 2**

Preparing your breakfast the night before is a clever way to help you make a sensible decision when you're hungry first thing in the morning. You just open the fridge and tuck into the goodness of oats, honey, and raspberries all ready to go. This is particularly good with a handful of chopped pistachios sprinkled over the top, but leave them out if you are being very strict with yourself.

1¼ cups rolled oats
1 teaspoon pumpkin pie spice
¾ cup 2% reduced-fat milk
½ cup raspberries, plus a few extra to serve
1 heaping tablespoon honey
¼ cup pistachios, roughly chopped,
   to serve (optional)

1. Put the rolled oats into a large bowl and sprinkle over the pumpkin pie spice. Pour in the milk and mix together well.

2. In a separate bowl, crush the raspberries and honey together with the back of a fork until roughly mashed.

3. Stir the raspberry mixture through the oats, then divide between two bowls or airtight containers, cover, and leave in the fridge overnight.

4. When ready to eat, remove the bowls from the fridge and top with a few extra raspberries and a sprinkle of chopped pistachios, if using.

| PER SERVING | |
| --- | --- |
| CALORIES | 299 |
| FAT (g) | 6.0 |
| SATURATED FAT (g) | 2.0 |
| CARBS (g) | 48.0 |
| SUGAR (g) | 15.0 |
| FIBER (g) | 5.0 |
| PROTEIN (g) | 10.0 |
| SODIUM (g) | 0.16 |

# SPINACH, TOMATO, AND FETA SCRAMBLED EGGS

**SERVES 4**

Feta is naturally lower in fat than many cheeses, and because the flavor is salty and intense, a little goes a long way. It also helps to keep the texture soft, as the eggs are less likely to overcook. These eggs are particularly good served with a little chili sauce. For active days, serve the scrambled eggs on whole-wheat or rye toast or with brown rice or quinoa, to make this a good breakfast for a training or race day.

Olive oil
12 cherry tomatoes, halved
Sea salt and freshly ground black pepper
3⅓ cups spinach leaves, washed and dried
8 eggs
3½ ounces feta cheese, crumbled

1. Place a large, deep skillet over medium heat and add a dash of oil. Once hot, put the tomatoes, cut side down, into the pan and season with salt and pepper. Cook for 3 to 4 minutes, until they start to color and caramelize slightly.

2. Turn the tomatoes over gently and put the spinach leaves on top. Cook for an additional 3 minutes, then stir gently to mix the spinach and tomatoes together.

3. Meanwhile, crack the eggs into a bowl, season with a pinch of pepper, and beat to combine.

4. Once the spinach has wilted, reduce the heat to medium-low, pour in the eggs, and add the crumbled feta. Gently cook, stirring regularly, until the eggs are mixed with the other ingredients and scrambled but not set.

5. Remove the pan from the heat, check the seasoning, and serve immediately.

| PER SERVING | |
| --- | --- |
| CALORIES | 239 |
| FAT (g) | 16.0 |
| SATURATED FAT (g) | 6.0 |
| CARBS (g) | 2.0 |
| SUGAR (g) | 2.0 |
| FIBER (g) | 1.0 |
| PROTEIN (g) | 19.0 |
| SODIUM (g) | 1.09 |

**VARIATIONS**
Herbs like dill, chives, parsley, and thyme are delicious in scrambled eggs, as are greens like chard, spring onions, and zucchini.

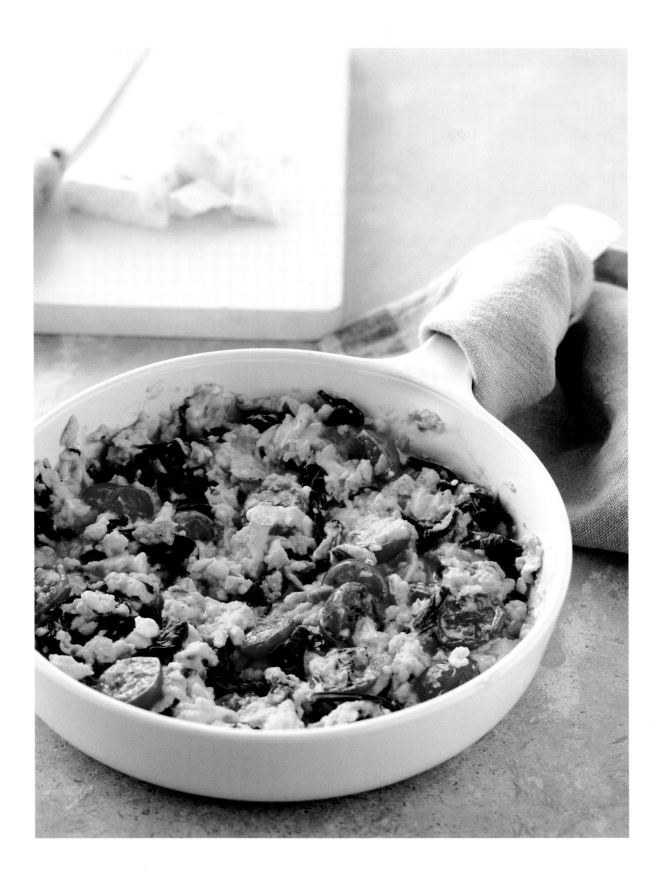

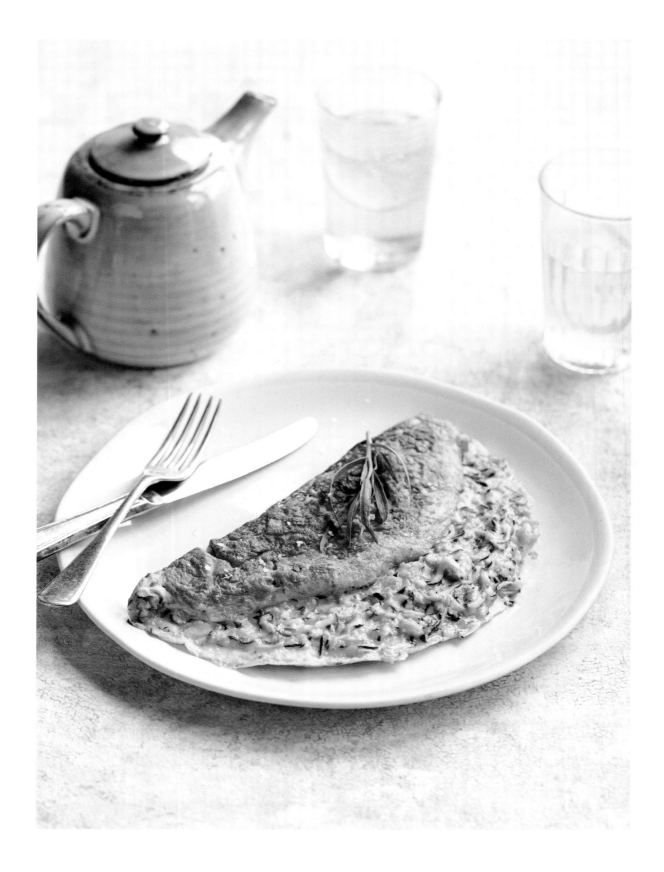

# ZUCCHINI OMELET

**SERVES 1**

When you're trying to lose weight, eating eggs for breakfast is a really good habit to get into. Recent research has found that people who start their day with two eggs eat fewer calories over the remainder of the day and lose more weight than those who eat a regular carb-loaded breakfast. This omelet is ideal for one person, and packing it with zucchini makes it even more filling and satisfying.

1 medium zucchini, grated
Olive oil
1 tarragon sprig, leaves finely chopped
2 eggs
Sea salt and freshly ground black pepper

1. Squeeze the grated zucchini to remove any excess water, then place a medium heavy-bottomed skillet over medium heat and add a dash of oil. When hot, add the grated zucchini and chopped tarragon and gently stir for 3 to 4 minutes, until the zucchini has softened.

2. Meanwhile, lightly beat the eggs with a fork and season with salt and pepper. Once the zucchini has softened, tip out any excess liquid, then return the pan to the heat and pour in the eggs. Quickly stir and shake the pan to distribute the egg, leave to cook for 3 to 4 minutes, until the egg is almost set, then remove from the heat.

3. With a heatproof spatula, loosen the sides of the omelet from the pan. Tip the pan slightly and coax the loosened edge down toward the bottom of the pan, folding the omelet in half. Next, slide or turn it out onto a serving plate and serve immediately.

**FOR ACTIVE DAYS**
If you want a great protein boost after a long workout, run, or race, make this omelet with three eggs instead of two, or add an extra egg white.

| PER SERVING | |
| --- | --- |
| CALORIES | 234 |
| FAT (g) | 16.0 |
| SATURATED FAT (g) | 4.0 |
| CARBS (g) | 3.0 |
| SUGAR (g) | 2.0 |
| FIBER (g) | 2.0 |
| PROTEIN (g) | 20.0 |
| SODIUM (g) | 0.52 |

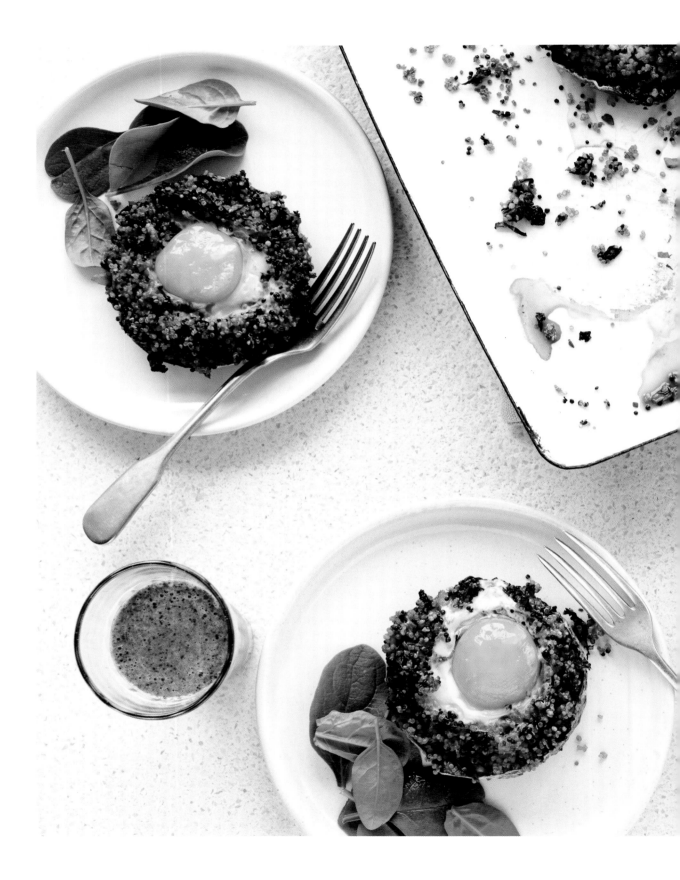

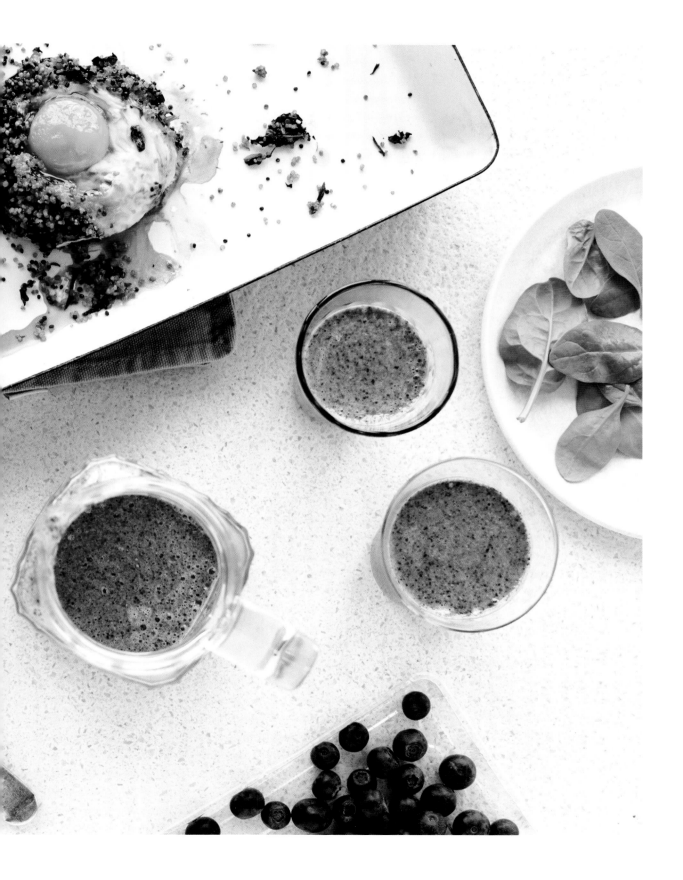

# QUINOA-STUFFED MUSHROOMS WITH BAKED EGGS

**SERVES 4**

Eggs are packed with protein and good-for-you fats, as well as B vitamins, vitamin D, zinc, and iron, and baking them inside whole mushrooms like this is really simple and very tasty. All the juices get absorbed by the mushrooms and quinoa and the slow-cooked eggs stay soft and runny. These are brilliant for a vegetarian breakfast or weekend brunch, or even lunch. It's one of those recipes that take a bit of time but not much effort, so you can get on with mixing up a virgin Mary to go with it.

4 large whole portobello mushrooms, stems removed and finely diced
Olive oil
Sea salt and freshly ground black pepper
1 garlic clove, peeled and finely chopped
3½ cups baby spinach, thinly sliced
1 cup cooked quinoa (from approximately ⅓ cup uncooked quinoa)
1 thyme sprig, leaves picked
4 small eggs

**1.** Preheat the oven to 350°F.

**2.** Place the mushrooms gill side down on a baking sheet, drizzle each one with a little olive oil, and season with a pinch of salt and pepper. Put the sheet into the oven and roast for 5 minutes.

**3.** Meanwhile, heat a skillet over medium heat and add a dash of olive oil. When hot, sauté the chopped mushroom stalks with a pinch of salt for 3 to 4 minutes, until softened. Add the garlic and spinach to the pan and sauté for 3 to 4 minutes, until wilted.

**4.** Stir in the cooked quinoa and thyme leaves.

**5.** Remove the mushrooms from the oven and turn them over so that the cups are facing upward. Flatten the gills down with the back of a spoon and fill with the quinoa and spinach mixture.

**6.** Create a small dip in the middle of each mushroom and carefully break an egg into each dip.

**7.** Put the sheet back into the oven for 10 to 12 minutes, until the whites are cooked through and the yolks are still runny. Serve immediately.

| PER SERVING | |
| --- | --- |
| CALORIES | 176 |
| FAT (g) | 9.0 |
| SATURATED FAT (g) | 2.0 |
| CARBS (g) | 10.0 |
| SUGAR (g) | 2.0 |
| FIBER (g) | 3.0 |
| PROTEIN (g) | 12.0 |
| SODIUM (g) | 0.26 |

# TOFU AND KALE SCRAMBLE
**SERVES 4**

I must admit that chefs don't always have good things to say about tofu! It can seem a bit spongy and tasteless, but spending time in LA where healthy eating is almost a religion, I have learned that there are ways of making it really tasty. And the nutritional benefits are worth overcoming any mental blocks for—it's full of protein, iron, and other nutrients and very low in fat at the same time.

1 tablespoon olive oil
1 small red onion, peeled and thinly sliced
Sea salt
7 ounces cremini mushrooms, sliced
1 garlic clove, peeled and finely chopped
5 ounces kale, roughly chopped
9 ounces firm tofu, drained, patted dry, and crumbled
½ to 1 tablespoon soy sauce
Pinch of turmeric
Dried chile flakes, to taste (optional)
Sea salt and freshly ground black pepper

1. Place a large skillet over medium heat and add the olive oil. Once hot, cook the onion with a pinch of salt for 5 to 6 minutes, until softened.

2. Add the mushrooms and cook for 3 to 4 minutes, until softened and beginning to lightly color. Add the garlic, stir, and cook for 1 more minute.

3. Stir in the chopped kale and add 2 tablespoons of water. Cover and leave for 5 minutes, or until the kale has completely wilted. Remove the lid and stir.

4. Mix in the crumbled tofu and add the soy sauce, turmeric, and chile flakes, if using. Season with salt and pepper, then stir-fry over medium-high heat for 2 to 3 minutes, until warmed through completely. Taste and add a little extra soy sauce and seasoning if needed.

5. Remove the pan from the heat and serve immediately.

**FOR ACTIVE DAYS**
Serve on whole-wheat or rye toast before exercise, or with Sweet Potato Chips (see page 241) the night before a big day.

| PER SERVING | |
| --- | --- |
| CALORIES | 159 |
| FAT (g) | 9.0 |
| SATURATED FAT (g) | 1.0 |
| CARBS (g) | 6.0 |
| SUGAR (g) | 1.0 |
| FIBER (g) | 2.0 |
| PROTEIN (g) | 13.0 |
| SODIUM (g) | 0.32 |

# LIGHT LUNCHES TO KEEP YOU ON TRACK

# CHICKEN AND QUINOA SATAY RICE PAPER ROLLS

**SERVES 4 (MAKES 16 ROLLS)**

Filled with lean chicken, quinoa, raw vegetables, and a punchy satay sauce, these are a great take on Vietnamese summer rolls and are a firm favorite in the Ramsay house. This combination is packed with protein, making these rolls ideal for the middle of the day because protein helps stave off midafternoon sugar cravings. You can swap the chicken for tuna, shrimp, or tofu, and vary the vegetables depending on what you have. The rolls will keep for a couple of days in the fridge, so they are ideal to make ahead to take to work or on a picnic.

½ cup quinoa, rinsed
1 skinless chicken breast
16 round rice paper wrappers
4 mint sprigs, leaves only
1 red pepper, seeded and thinly sliced
1 zucchini, julienned
1 ripe avocado, peeled, pitted, and sliced
2 spring onions, thinly sliced
Juice of 1 lime

**FOR THE SATAY SAUCE**

2 tablespoons sugar-free peanut butter, smooth or crunchy
1½ teaspoons soy sauce
1 teaspoon agave syrup or runny honey
Pinch of dried chile flakes, or to taste
1 teaspoon rice vinegar
½ teaspoon grated fresh ginger

**CONTINUED ON PAGE 130**

| PER SERVING | |
| --- | --- |
| CALORIES | 387 |
| FAT (g) | 13.0 |
| SATURATED FAT (g) | 3.0 |
| CARBS (g) | 49.0 |
| SUGAR (g) | 6.0 |
| FIBER (g) | 5.0 |
| PROTEIN (g) | 17.0 |
| SODIUM (g) | 1.52 |

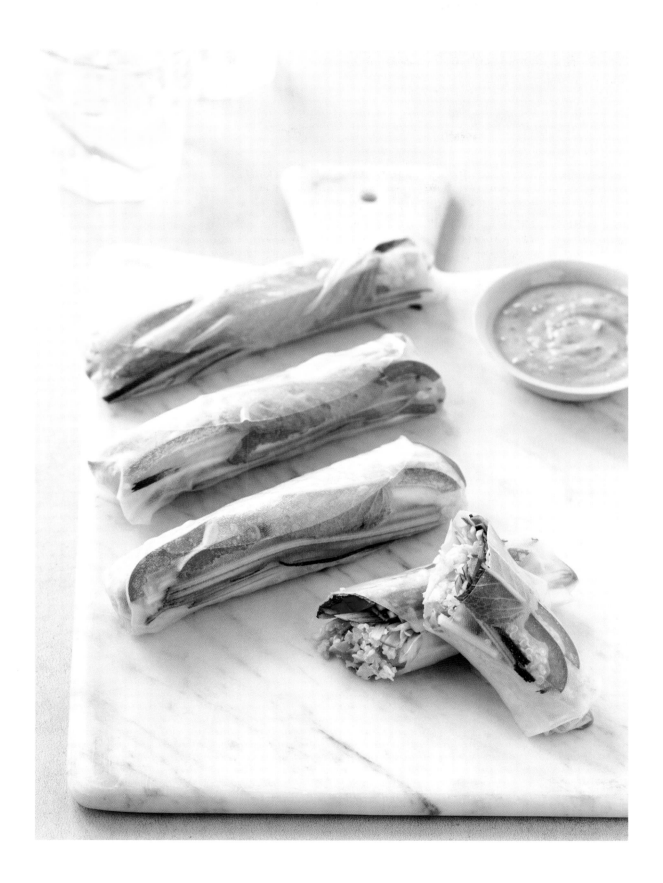

CONTINUED FROM PAGE 128

1. Cook the quinoa according to the package instructions. Set aside to cool.

2. Poach the chicken breast in a medium saucepan of simmering water for 15 minutes. Once cooked, remove the breast from the water and leave to cool.

3. In the meantime, make the satay sauce: Mix together all the ingredients in a small bowl with a fork and thin with a teaspoon of warm water at a time until you reach a dipping consistency (approximately 5 to 7 teaspoons of water). The mixture will look like it's splitting at first, but if you slowly mix it with a fork, it will come together and thicken. Taste and adjust the flavors as necessary.

4. Once the chicken has cooled, tear the breast into thin strips.

5. To make the rolls, place a rice paper wrapper in a bowl of warm water for 10 to 15 seconds, until soft and pliable. Place it on a cutting board, then put a mint leaf in the center and top with a couple of pieces of red pepper, zucchini, avocado, and spring onion. Add a tablespoon of the cooked quinoa and a couple of strips of chicken, then drizzle a little lime juice over the top.

6. Fold the sides of the rice paper over the filling, then, rolling from the bottom, using your fingers to keep the filling tightly encased, roll up tightly into a spring roll shape and repeat with the remaining ingredients.

7. Serve the rolls with the dipping sauce on the side.

**GOOD TO KNOW**
Rice paper is low in fat and calories and therefore a better lunch option than bread when you are trying to lose weight. Raw vegetables add color and crunch as well as lots of nutrients that are lost when they are cooked.

# LENTIL, CARROT, AND CILANTRO SOUP

**SERVES 4**

When you are trying to lose weight, soup is like a secret weapon . . . it's low in calories but more filling than eating the same ingredients "dry," due to the water content. This warming lentil soup is comforting and wholesome and will help keep you on track, as it keeps hunger at bay for much longer than salad. It's important to "cook out" the garam masala to get the best flavor, so don't add the grated carrots until the aromas from the spices are released and the room is full of wonderful smells.

2 tablespoons olive oil
1 red onion, peeled and diced
1 garlic clove, peeled and roughly chopped
1¼-inch piece of fresh ginger, peeled and roughly chopped
½ bunch of cilantro, leaves picked and stems reserved
1 tablespoon garam masala
1 pound carrots, grated
1 cup red lentils
1½ quarts vegetable stock
1 red chile, seeded and thinly sliced

**TO SERVE**
¼ cup low-fat yogurt
1 lemon, quartered

1. Place a large saucepan over medium–high heat and add the oil. When hot, add the onion, garlic, and ginger.

2. Finely chop the cilantro stems and add them to the pan. Sweat the ingredients for 5 minutes.

3. Sprinkle in the garam masala and cook for 30 seconds, stirring almost constantly, then add the grated carrots and stir well.

4. Add the lentils and stock and bring to a boil. Reduce the heat and simmer for about 35 minutes, until all the ingredients are completely soft.

5. Roughly chop the cilantro leaves, then serve the soup in warmed bowls, topped with a sprinkle of cilantro and chile and a good dollop of yogurt, with a wedge of lemon on the side.

| PER SERVING | |
| --- | --- |
| CALORIES | 305 |
| FAT (g) | 8.0 |
| SATURATED FAT (g) | 1.0 |
| CARBS (g) | 40.0 |
| SUGAR (g) | 15.0 |
| FIBER (g) | 11.0 |
| PROTEIN (g) | 13.0 |
| SODIUM (g) | 1.08 |

# HARISSA HUMMUS WITH CARROT ON RYE
**SERVES 4**

Eating more beans is really helpful when you are trying to lose weight, because they give you lots of filling fiber and protein without too many calories. Strong flavors help, too, and I often reach for chile in some form or another, not least because it is said to raise your metabolism and help burn fat. Harissa is a hot, aromatic chile paste from North Africa that livens up marinades, rubs, dressings, and pasta sauces. You could also blend some leafy vegetables like spinach or chard through the hummus for added greens.

1 (15-ounce) can white beans, such as cannellini, drained and rinsed
1 garlic clove, peeled and roughly chopped
Juice of ½ lemon
½ teaspoon ground cumin
½ tablespoon harissa paste, or to taste
1 tablespoon tahini
Sea salt and freshly ground black pepper
1 tablespoon extra virgin olive oil

**TO SERVE**
8 slices of rye or pumpernickel bread
3 carrots, grated
Chopped chives

1. Put the drained beans, garlic, lemon juice, cumin, harissa paste, tahini, and a little salt and pepper into a small food processor and process until almost smooth but still with a little texture.

2. With the motor running, slowly pour in the olive oil. Taste and adjust the seasoning as needed. Add more harissa paste if you like it a little hotter.

3. Spread the hummus on the 8 slices of bread. Add the grated carrot to 4 of the slices, sprinkle with chives, and put the other 4 slices on top. Slice the sandwiches in half and eat immediately, or wrap in plastic wrap to take with you.

| PER SERVING | |
| --- | --- |
| CALORIES | 260 |
| FAT (g) | 7.0 |
| SATURATED FAT (g) | 1.0 |
| CARBS (g) | 34.0 |
| SUGAR (g) | 6.0 |
| FIBER (g) | 10.0 |
| PROTEIN (g) | 10.0 |
| SODIUM (g) | 0.82 |

**GOOD TO KNOW**
As many of the nutrients in carrots are found in the skin or just under it, it makes sense not to peel them, but make sure you give them a really good scrub before serving them raw.

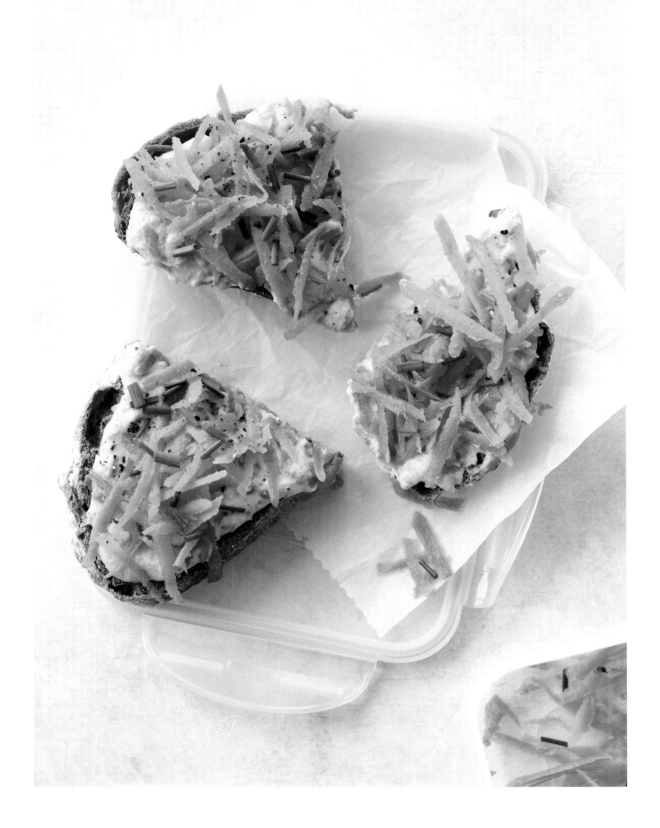

# EGG "MAYONNAISE" AND SPINACH SANDWICH

**SERVES 4**

Lose the real mayonnaise and you turn this into a much lighter choice than a store-bought egg salad sandwich. You can still add all the traditional mayo flavorings such as a squeeze of lemon juice or vinegar and a little dash of mustard, but the base is much healthier than the oil and egg yolks of a standard mayonnaise. This is delicious with the addition of finely diced pickles, too.

6 eggs
¼ cup regular or Greek yogurt
1½ teaspoons cider vinegar
1 teaspoon Dijon mustard
Squeeze of lemon juice
2 celery stalks, finely diced
3 dill sprigs, finely chopped
Sea salt and freshly ground black pepper
8 slices of whole-wheat bread
4 handfuls of baby spinach leaves, washed

1. Bring a large saucepan of water to a boil and gently add the eggs. Boil for 10 minutes, then remove them from the water and put them into a bowl of cold water with ice until cooled.

2. Meanwhile, put the yogurt, vinegar, mustard, lemon juice, diced celen, and chopped dill into a large mixing bowl. Season with salt and pepper and stir everything together until well combined.

3. Once the eggs are cooled, peel and dice them or mash with a fork, then add to the yogurt mixture. Mix everything together. Taste and adjust the seasoning as necessary.

4. Divide the egg mixture among the 8 slices of bread and top 4 of the slices with a handful of spinach. Place the remaining slices on top and cut the sandwiches in half to serve, or wrap in plastic wrap and store in the fridge for later.

| PER SERVING | |
|---|---|
| CALORIES | 399 |
| FAT (g) | 15.0 |
| SATURATED FAT (g) | 6.0 |
| CARBS (g) | 26.0 |
| SUGAR (g) | 4.0 |
| FIBER (g) | 5.0 |
| PROTEIN (g) | 22.0 |
| SODIUM (g) | 1.2 |

# BROWN RICE SUSHI HAND ROLLS

**SERVES 4 (MAKES 8 HAND ROLLS)**

I absolutely love Japanese food, and it is always a great choice when trying to lose weight because the ingredients and cooking methods are naturally low in fat and nutrient-rich. What's more, the sauces and seasonings are strong and satisfying—diet food should never be boring. Hand rolls look impressive but are actually quite easy to put together. I've used smoked salmon in this recipe because it's easy to get ahold of, but if you have access to a brilliant fishmonger and really fresh, sushi-grade fish, then go down the more traditional route and make these with raw salmon or tuna.

½ cup brown sushi rice or short-grain brown rice
1½ tablespoons mirin
1½ tablespoons rice vinegar
Sea salt
4 sheets of nori seaweed
5 ounces sliced smoked salmon, torn into
   bite-size pieces
1 ripe avocado, peeled, pitted, and cubed
½ cucumber, cut into thick strips
2 tablespoons sesame seeds, black or tan
½ cup sushi ginger
Soy sauce, to serve

**CONTINUED ON PAGE 137**

**GOOD TO KNOW**
Seaweed like nori is very nutrient dense and is especially valued for its high mineral content, including iodine, which is essential for a healthy metabolism.

| PER SERVING | |
| --- | --- |
| CALORIES | 299 |
| FAT (g) | 14.0 |
| SATURATED FAT (g) | 3.0 |
| CARBS (g) | 27.0 |
| SUGAR (g) | 3.0 |
| FIBER (g) | 4.0 |
| PROTEIN (g) | 14.0 |
| SODIUM (g) | 1.40 |

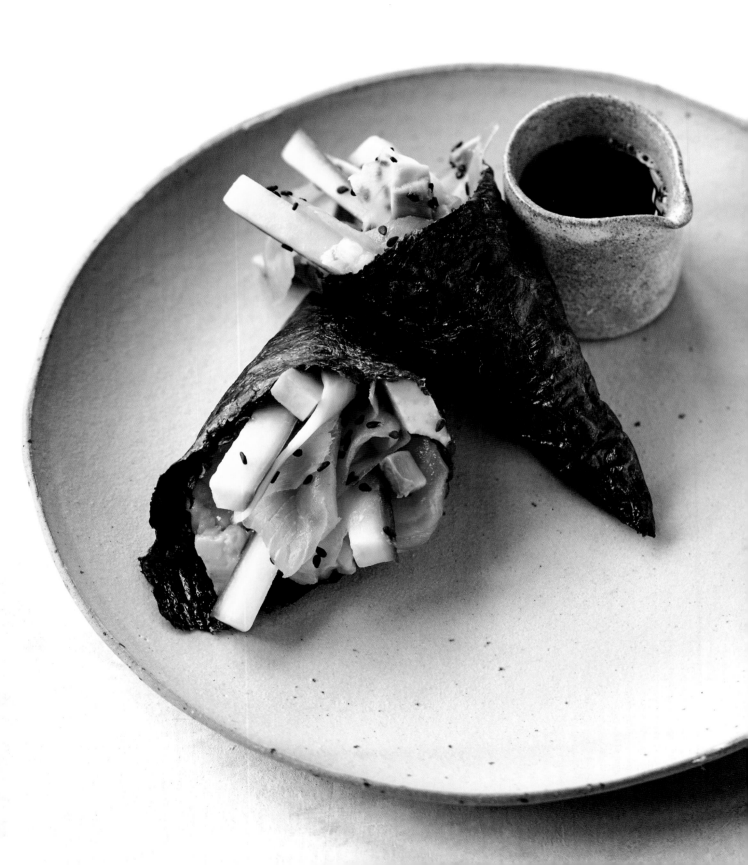

CONTINUED FROM PAGE 135

1. Rinse the rice really well in a sieve under cold running water until the water runs clear.

2. Put the rice into a medium saucepan with a tight-fitting lid and pour over 1 cup of water. Bring to a simmer, then reduce the heat to low. Put the lid on and leave the pan for 30 minutes over low heat without removing the lid, or until all the water has been absorbed and the rice is tender. Remove the pan from the heat and leave to stand for 10 minutes with the lid still on.

3. After 10 minutes, spread the rice on a clean baking sheet and sprinkle over the mirin, rice vinegar, and a couple of pinches of salt. Mix the rice together to make sure everything is coated and spread out to cool at room temperature.

4. Once the rice has cooled and you are ready to assemble the hand rolls, cut the nori sheets in half, then fill a small bowl with warm water. Place one piece of seaweed on a board with the long side facing toward you. Add 1 tablespoon of rice to the middle of the right-hand half of the sheet. Wet your hands and press the rice down gently to flatten it. Place a couple of pieces of salmon on the rice and top with avocado, cucumber, a sprinkling of sesame seeds, and a couple of pieces of sushi ginger. The top right corner will be the open end, so place the cucumber with one end at that corner to make it easier to roll.

5. Take the bottom right corner of the nori sheet and fold it over so that it covers the filling and is now at the top left corner of the right half of the nori sheet. You should have an opening where the top right corner was. Now, with your fingers securing the nori sheet covering the filling, roll tightly toward the empty left-hand side of the sheet to create a tight cone shape. The bottom left corner of the right-hand half of the sheet will be the point from which you pivot the cone. Wet the edge of the nori sheet with your fingers and stick it to the cone, securing the nori tightly. Repeat with the remaining sheets and filling.

6. Serve the hand rolls with soy sauce on the side.

**VARIATION**
If you can't get hold of brown sushi rice or short-grain brown rice, then replace with white sushi rice. However, this rice will not be as sticky, so make sure to wrap your hand rolls tightly to keep the contents from spilling out.

# CHICKEN AND KALE CAESAR SALAD

**SERVES 4**

Massaging kale sounds like a crazy thing to do, but it actually tenderizes the leaves, making them soft enough to eat without having to cook them. You can also dress this salad up to two days in advance, which will tenderize the leaves further. If you miss the croutons in a classic Caesar salad, try sprinkling Crunchy Chickpeas (page 99) over the top instead.

1 bunch kale, stalks removed and leaves torn
Sea salt and freshly ground black pepper
Olive oil
2 skinless chicken breasts, butterflied
1 head chicory, leaves separated

**FOR THE DRESSING**
1 garlic clove, peeled and roughly chopped
4 anchovy fillets, drained and roughly chopped
½ teaspoon Dijon mustard
2 tablespoons grated Parmesan cheese, plus extra to serve (optional)
Juice of ¼ to ½ lemon, to taste
1 tablespoon extra virgin olive oil
⅔ cup plain yogurt

1. Put the torn kale into a large mixing bowl, season with salt and pepper, and drizzle with the olive oil. Rub the oil and seasoning into the kale leaves for a few minutes to help tenderize the leaves, then leave for 30 minutes while you prepare the rest of the salad.

2. Heat a grill pan over medium–high heat. Rub the butterflied chicken breasts with a little olive oil and season with salt and pepper. Place on the pan and cook for 3 to 4 minutes on each side, until just cooked through. Remove the chicken and leave to rest.

3. Meanwhile, make the dressing: Put all the ingredients into a blender and blitz until smooth. Taste and adjust the seasoning, adding a little more lemon juice if needed.

4. Once the chicken has cooled and the kale is tenderized, toss the kale and chicory with the dressing, mixing really well to coat the leaves. Slice the chicken, place it on top, then grate over a little Parmesan, if using.

| PER SERVING | |
| --- | --- |
| CALORIES | 241 |
| FAT (g) | 12.0 |
| SATURATED FAT (g) | 3.0 |
| CARBS (g) | 5.0 |
| SUGAR (g) | 4.0 |
| FIBER (g) | 4.0 |
| PROTEIN (g) | 28.0 |
| SODIUM (g) | 0.92 |

**HOW TO SOFTEN KALE**
If you don't have time to massage and marinate the kale leaves, you can also blanch them very briefly in boiling water, then refresh them in iced water and dry thoroughly.

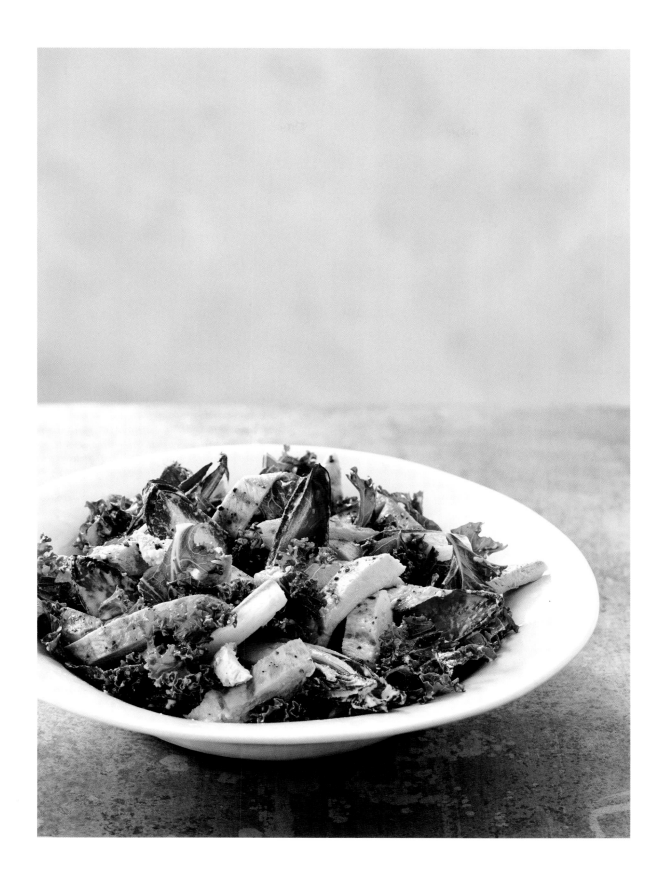

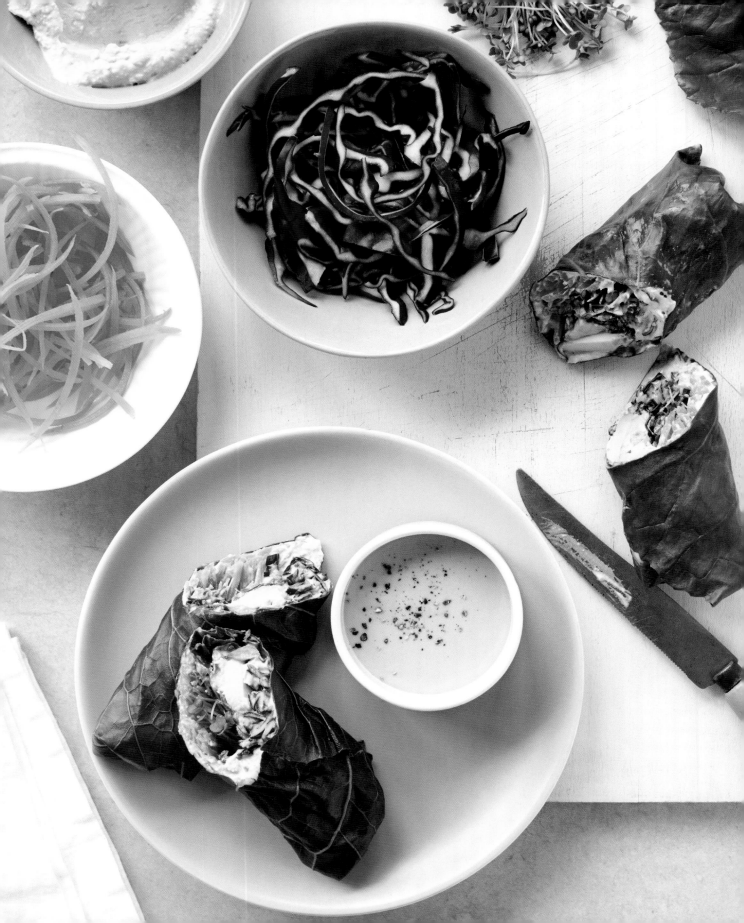

# COLLARD GREEN WRAPS
**SERVES 4 (MAKES 8 WRAPS)**

Using collard green leaves to make wraps is an ingenious way of upping your vegetable intake. They have a lovely crunchy texture and work surprisingly well in place of a tortilla or rice paper wrapper. You could also use Savoy cabbage leaves, or swap the leaves for whole-wheat wraps or tortillas if you are trying to get in some carbs before exercising.

**FOR THE DRESSING/DIPPING SAUCE**
¼ cup tahini
1 tablespoon soy sauce
2 teaspoons maple syrup or runny honey
Juice of 1 lime
Sea salt and freshly ground black pepper

**FOR THE WRAPS**
8 large collard green leaves
1 cup hummus
2 carrots, grated
¼ small red cabbage, very finely shredded
1 ripe avocado, peeled, pitted, and sliced
2 cups radish or other sprouts or microgreens

1. To make the dressing/dipping sauce, put all the ingredients into a bowl with a pinch of salt and pepper. Mix well until completely combined, then add warm water 1 teaspoon at a time, mixing after each addition until you reach a drizzling/dipping consistency.

2. Fill a medium skillet three-quarters full with hot water and bring to a simmer. Cut the woody stem from the bottom of each collard green leaf and trim the interior stems so the leaves are pliable, leaving as much of the leaf as possible intact. Dip each leaf, one at a time, into the hot water for 10 seconds, or until wilted and bright green in color. Remove and set aside.

3. Spread the leaves out on a board. Divide the hummus among the leaves and spread it out.

4. Arrange a little grated carrot, shredded red cabbage, sliced avocado, and sprouts in the middle of each leaf. Drizzle each pile of vegetables with a little dressing, then fold the sides of the leaves inward over the filling and roll up from the bottom, enclosing the mixture completely.

5. Place the wraps, edge side down, on a board and slice them diagonally through the middle, then serve with the dipping sauce in a bowl on the side.

**HOW TO SOFTEN COLLARD LEAVES**
If you don't have time to blanch the collard leaves, you can put them in the microwave for 10 to 12 seconds to soften them.

| PER SERVING | |
| --- | --- |
| CALORIES | 331 |
| FAT (g) | 23.0 |
| SATURATED FAT (g) | 4.0 |
| CARBS (g) | 17.0 |
| SUGAR (g) | 8.0 |
| FIBER (g) | 9.0 |
| PROTEIN (g) | 9.0 |
| SODIUM (g) | 0.90 |

# LEAN SUPPERS AND SIDES

# MEXICAN SHRIMP COCKTAIL

**SERVES 4**

The Mexican version of shrimp cocktail is made with a tangy tomato-based sauce spiked with lime and chile. It's quite different and much more refreshing—my family are total converts. Serve as a starter with Pita Chips (page 266) for added crunch, or unsalted tortilla chips if you aren't going for lean.

1½ tablespoons ketchup
Juice of ½ orange
1 teaspoon Worcestershire sauce
Juice of 1 lime
¼ cup roughly chopped cilantro leaves and stems
4 medium tomatoes, diced
1 small white onion, peeled and finely diced
1 cucumber, finely diced
Sea salt and freshly ground black pepper
14 ounces cooked shrimp, peeled and deveined if necessary
1 ripe avocado, peeled, pitted, and diced

**TO SERVE**
1 lime, quartered
Mexican hot sauce, such as Cholula (optional)

**1.** In a large mixing bowl, combine the ketchup, orange juice, Worcestershire sauce, and lime juice and mix until thoroughly combined. Add the cilantro leaves and stems, tomatoes, onion, and cucumber and mix well. Season with a little salt and pepper.

**2.** Stir in the shrimp and coat with the sauce. Taste and adjust the seasoning as necessary.

**3.** Serve the shrimp cocktail in cocktail glasses or small bowls, with the avocado sprinkled over the top and a lime wedge on the side. This is delicious with a few drops of Mexican hot sauce on top.

| PER SERVING | |
| --- | --- |
| CALORIES | 185 |
| FAT (g) | 8.0 |
| SATURATED FAT (g) | 2.0 |
| CARBS (g) | 8.0 |
| SUGAR (g) | 7.0 |
| FIBER (g) | 4.0 |
| PROTEIN (g) | 19.0 |
| SODIUM (g) | 1.79 |

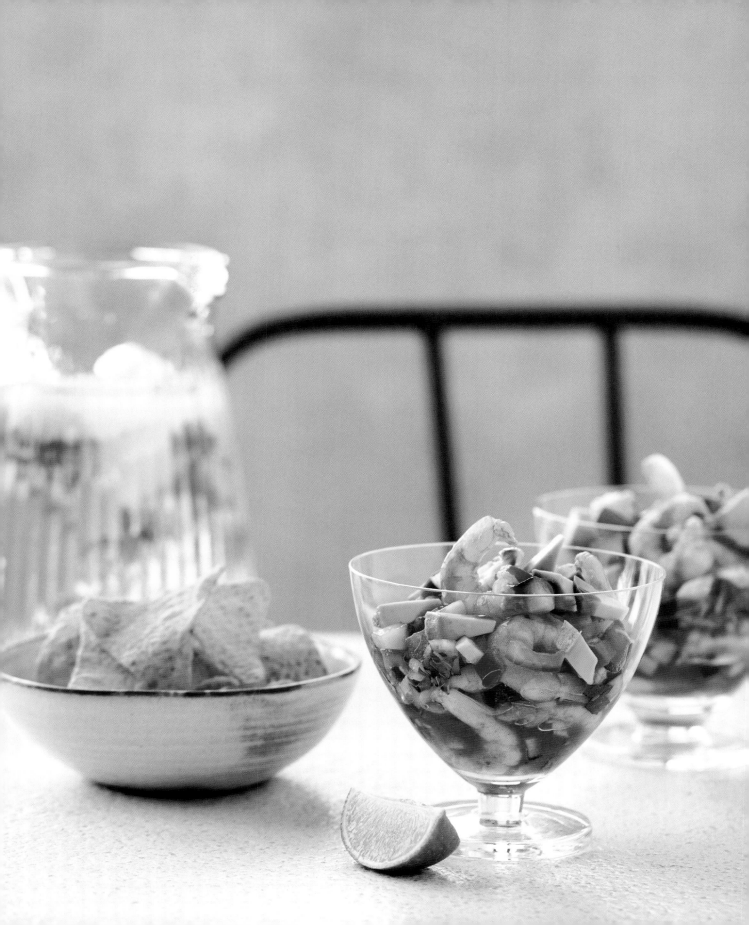

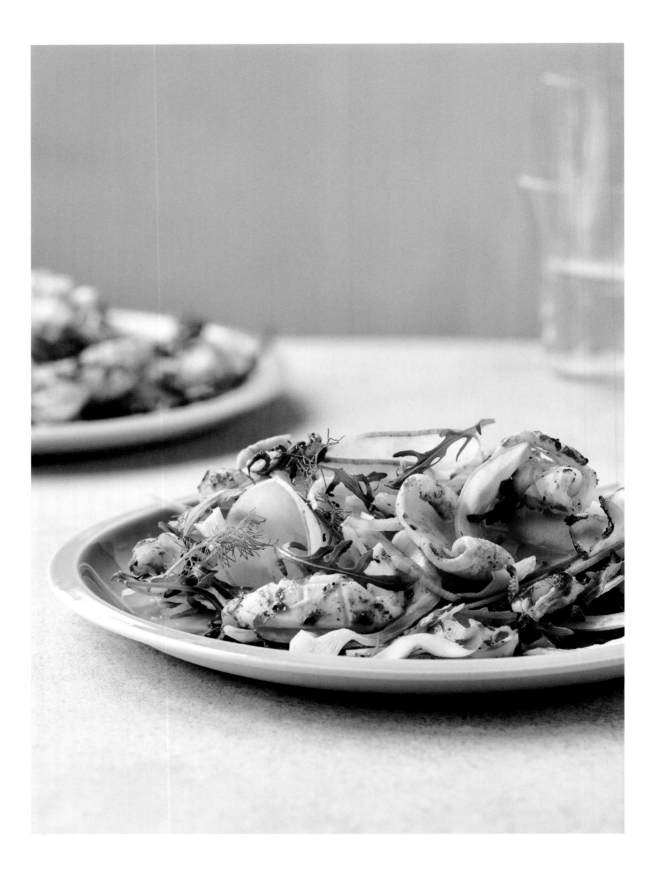

# GRILLED SQUID, FENNEL, AND APPLE SALAD

**SERVES 4**

Squid should be cooked either very fast or very slow—anything in between and you will feel like you're tucking into a plate of rubber bands. So when I say cook for 1 minute on each side, that's exactly what I mean . . . this should be just long enough for the flesh to turn opaque but still stay tender. When you're not trying hard to keep your meals lean, a little chorizo added to this salad is absolutely delicious.

4 medium squid (about 14 ounces), cleaned
Olive oil, for drizzling
1 teaspoon smoked paprika
Sea salt and freshly ground black pepper
1 large fennel bulb
1 large tart apple, such as
    Granny Smith, cored
Juice of 1 lemon
5 ounces (7½ cups) arugula leaves
2 mint sprigs, leaves roughly torn
Sherry vinegar

1. Slice the squid tubes open and lightly score one side in a diamond pattern before slicing each tube into 6 pieces. Cut any large tentacles into smaller bite-size pieces and place everything in a medium mixing bowl. Drizzle with olive oil and sprinkle over the smoked paprika and a pinch of salt and pepper. Toss to make sure everything is coated with smoked paprika and set aside.

2. Meanwhile, thinly slice the fennel and apple, ideally on a mandoline or with a very sharp knife. Put the slices into a bowl of cold water with the lemon juice to prevent them from turning brown.

3. Heat a grill pan over high heat. Once hot, add the squid, in batches if necessary, and cook for about 1 minute on each side, until lightly charred and just cooked through.

4. Drain the fennel and apple and pat dry with a clean dish towel or paper towels. Put the slices onto a serving plate and mix in the arugula and the torn mint leaves. Drizzle with a little olive oil, sherry vinegar, and a pinch of salt and pepper, then place the hot squid on top and sprinkle with a few extra dots of sherry vinegar. Serve immediately.

**HOW TO BARBECUE SQUID**
You could also grill the squid on the barbecue for a more charred, smoky flavor. Cut the flesh into slightly bigger pieces so that they don't fall through the gaps in the grill, and cook for 1 minute on each side.

| PER SERVING | |
|---|---|
| CALORIES | 180 |
| FAT (g) | 8.0 |
| SATURATED FAT (g) | 1.0 |
| CARBS (g) | 6.0 |
| SUGAR (g) | 6.0 |
| FIBER (g) | 5.0 |
| PROTEIN (g) | 18.0 |
| SODIUM (g) | 0.34 |

# SALMON CEVICHE WITH GRAPEFRUIT, AVOCADO, AND MINT

**SERVES 4**

This salmon ceviche is a simple but smart dish to serve when you are watching your weight. It is low in calories, but the combination of flavors is bold and satisfying; and because the fish isn't exposed to heat, it retains all of the valuable omega-3 fats that might otherwise be damaged during cooking. The bitter grapefruit juice goes brilliantly with the salmon, but you could swap it for any other meaty white fish, too—just make sure that whatever fish you choose, it's as fresh as possible.

1 pink or red grapefruit
14 ounces salmon fillet, skin and pinbones removed, thinly sliced
1 small shallot, peeled and finely diced
3½ ounces radishes, trimmed and thinly sliced
Sea salt
1 ripe avocado, peeled, pitted, and diced
5 mint sprigs, leaves roughly torn

**1.** Cut the grapefruit in half horizontally, then juice one of the halves. Remove the segments from the second half—do this over a bowl to collect any juices.

**2.** Put the sliced salmon, grapefruit juice and segments, diced shallot, and radishes into a large mixing bowl and season with couple of pinches of salt. Toss well to mix and leave to stand for 10 minutes or up to 30 minutes (see tip on page 76).

**3.** When ready to serve, transfer the ceviche to a serving plate or shallow bowl. Fold in the avocado and sprinkle over the torn mint leaves. Taste and adjust the seasoning as necessary, and serve immediately.

| PER SERVING | |
| --- | --- |
| CALORIES | 270 |
| FAT (g) | 17.0 |
| SATURATED FAT (g) | 4.0 |
| CARBS (g) | 4.0 |
| SUGAR (g) | 3.0 |
| FIBER (g) | 3.0 |
| PROTEIN (g) | 23.0 |
| SODIUM (g) | 0.14 |

**FOR ACTIVE DAYS**
If you are not counting calories, serve the ceviche with Melba toast, rye or pumpernickel bread, or the Pita Chips on page 266.

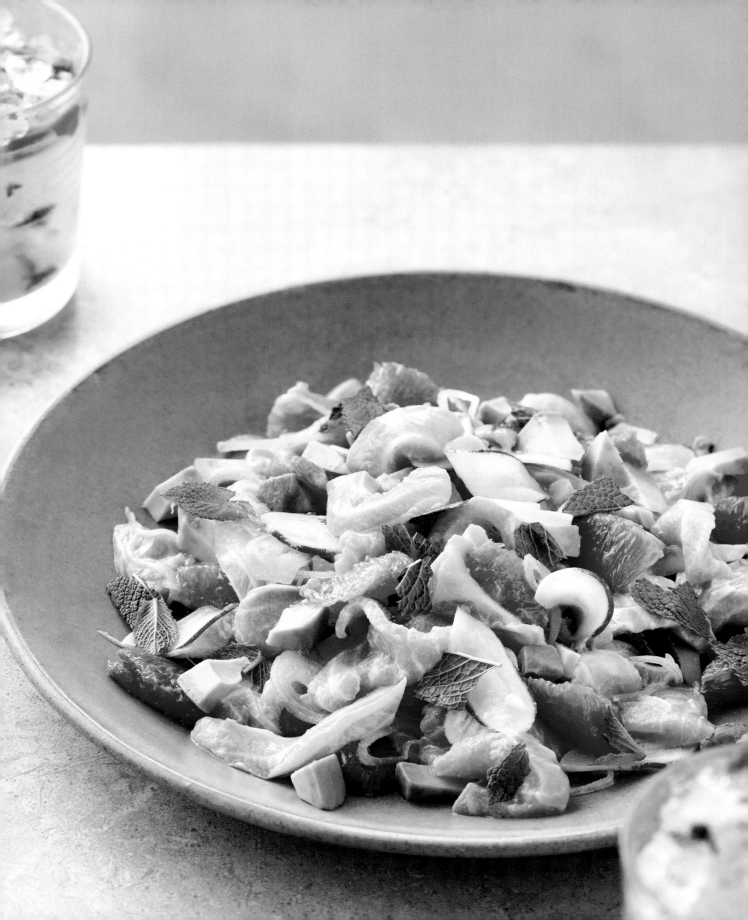

# EDAMAME, FAVA BEAN, AND PEA SOUP

**SERVES 4**

Edamame, fava beans, peas, and eggs are all excellent sources of protein, making this a really filling soup that will keep you satisfied long after you have eaten it—which means no hankering for off-limits snacks. Use frozen beans and peas for this recipe so you don't have to spend time shelling them before cooking.

1 tablespoon canola oil
1 large onion, peeled and diced
2 celery stalks, trimmed and diced
1 medium potato, peeled and diced
2 thyme sprigs, leaves only, plus a few extra leaves to garnish
1 quart chicken stock
7 ounces fave beans, shelled
5 ounces edamame, shelled
4 eggs
⅔ cup peas
1 red chile, seeded and thinly sliced
1½ teaspoons black sesame seeds

**1.** Place a large saucepan over medium heat and add the canola oil. When hot, add the onion, celery, potato, and thyme leaves and cook for 8 minutes, stirring regularly.

**2.** Pour in the stock and bring to a boil. Simmer for 10 minutes, then add the fava beans and edamame and simmer for an additional 10 minutes.

**3.** Meanwhile, bring a large saucepan of water to a boil, then reduce the heat and poach the eggs for 3 minutes, or until the whites have set but the yolks are still runny (see below).

**4.** When the beans are cooked, add the peas and bring to a boil again. Blitz the ingredients with a blender.

**5.** Divide the soup among four warmed bowls, slide an egg into each one, then sprinkle with red chile slices, black sesame seeds, and a few extra thyme leaves before serving.

| PER SERVING | |
| --- | --- |
| CALORIES | 334 |
| FAT (g) | 14.0 |
| SATURATED FAT (g) | 3.0 |
| CARBS (g) | 22.0 |
| SUGAR (g) | 7.0 |
| FIBER (g) | 11.0 |
| PROTEIN (g) | 25.0 |
| SODIUM (g) | 0.89 |

## HOW TO POACH AN EGG

Bring a large pan of water to a boil with a little splash of vinegar, then reduce to a gentle bubble. Use a whisk to stir the water in a circle to create a whirlpool. Crack the egg into a tea cup and slip it into the center of the circulating water. Poach for 3 minutes, or until the egg floats to the surface, then remove from the pan and drain on paper towels before serving.

# TAMARIND SHRIMP

**SERVES 4**

Tamarind has a sweet but tart flavor that goes really well with shrimp and fish. Here I am balancing the sourness with salty fish sauce and sweet agave syrup to make a distinct sweet-and-sour sauce that is popular across Southeast Asia. These shrimp are lip-smackingly good as a light starter or served with brown rice and Asian greens for a main dish.

1½ cups brown rice
3 tablespoons tamarind paste or watered-down tamarind block (see below)
1 tablespoon fish sauce, or to taste
1 tablespoon agave syrup, or to taste
1 tablespoon coconut oil or cooking oil of your choice
1 shallot, peeled and thinly sliced
2 garlic cloves, peeled and thinly sliced
4 heads bok choy
14 ounces large shrimp, patted dry
½ cup cilantro, roughly chopped

**CONTINUED ON PAGE 153**

**HOW TO PREPARE TAMARIND**
To water down a block of tamarind, soak it in a little hot water, remove the seeds, and mash it well to create a thick juice.

| PER SERVING | |
| --- | --- |
| CALORIES | 434 |
| FAT (g) | 7.0 |
| SATURATED FAT (g) | 3.0 |
| CARBS (g) | 64.0 |
| SUGAR (g) | 10.0 |
| FIBER (g) | 5.0 |
| PROTEIN (g) | 26.0 |
| SODIUM (g) | 1.43 |

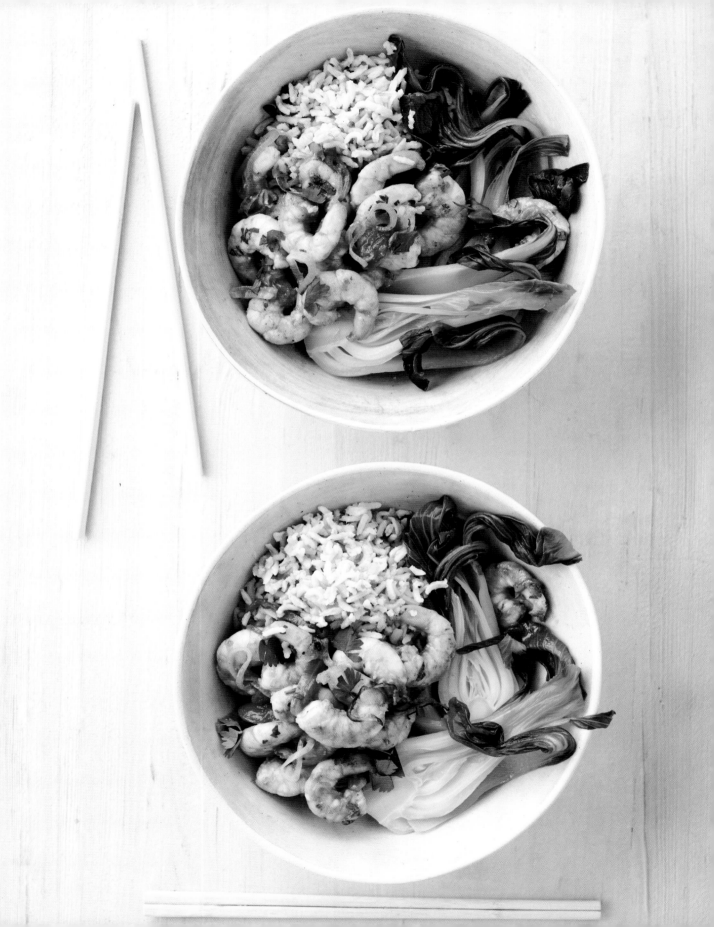

1. Rinse the rice really well in a sieve under cold running water until the water runs clear.

2. Put the rice into a medium saucepan with a tight-fitting lid and pour over 2½ cups of water. Bring to a simmer, then reduce the heat to low. Put the lid on and leave the pan for 30 minutes over low heat without removing the lid, or until all the water has been absorbed and the rice is tender.

3. Mix the tamarind, fish sauce, and agave syrup together in a separate small saucepan and place over low heat. Stir until completely combined. Taste and adjust the sweetness and saltiness as necessary. Set aside.

4. When the rice is cooked, remove the pan from the heat and leave to stand for 10 minutes with the lid on.

5. Place a wok or a large skillet over high heat and add the coconut oil. Once hot, cook the shallot and garlic for 4 to 5 minutes, until softened and turning slightly golden on the edges.

6. Meanwhile, slice the bok choy in half lengthwise and cook in a large pan of salted boiling water for 3 minutes, or until wilted.

7. Once the shallots are softened, add the shrimp to the pan and stir-fry for 2 minutes, then pour over the tamarind sauce. Stir so the shrimp are well coated, then cook for an additional 2 to 3 minutes, until the shrimp are cooked through and the sauce is thick enough to coat them.

8. When ready to serve, remove the lid from the rice pan and fluff up the rice with a fork.

9. Divide the rice, shrimp, and bok choy among four plates or bowls and garnish with the chopped cilantro.

# SEARED TUNA AND VEGETABLE SKEWERS WITH WASABI DIPPING SAUCE

**SERVES 4**

Despite being an oily fish, tuna can dry out very easily, so don't overcook these skewers—the cubes of fish should still be a little pink in the center. You can try other vegetables here—sugar snap peas or zucchini chunks would also be delicious, as would adding slivers of pickled sushi ginger between the tuna chunks. Pile up the skewers on a large plate or board and serve with the dipping sauce for everyone to help themselves, or plate them with some brown rice and Asian Slaw (page 156).

4 tuna steaks (approximately 5 ounces each), cut into 1-inch cubes
2 tablespoons soy sauce
1 small bunch of asparagus, trimmed
Sea salt
Neutral oil, such as peanut

**FOR THE WASABI DIPPING SAUCE**
1 to 2 teaspoons wasabi powder, or 2 teaspoons wasabi paste, to taste (see below)
3 tablespoons soy sauce
1 tablespoon runny honey, or ½ tablespoon agave syrup
1 teaspoon toasted sesame oil
1 tablespoon rice vinegar

1. Put the tuna cubes into a bowl and pour over the soy sauce. Massage gently into the tuna and leave to marinate.

2. Blanch the asparagus in a large pan of salted boiling water for 2 minutes. Remove from the pan and refresh immediately in cold water.

3. Slice the asparagus diagonally into 1¼-inch-long pieces.

4. Mix together the ingredients for the wasabi dipping sauce, starting with 1 teaspoon of the wasabi powder or paste. Taste and add more if you like a stronger wasabi flavor and a little more punch.

5. Place a grill pan or large skillet over medium heat.

6. Thread the tuna cubes and asparagus alternately onto skewers (if using bamboo skewers, soak them in water for 20 minutes beforehand).

7. Drizzle a little oil on a plate and roll each skewer in the oil, then place on the hot pan. Cook for 2 to 3 minutes on each side, until lightly marked but still pink in the middle (you may have to do this in batches, depending on the size of the pan).

8. Serve the skewers warm or at room temperature, with the dipping sauce on the side.

| PER SERVING | |
| --- | --- |
| CALORIES | 241 |
| FAT (g) | 5.0 |
| SATURATED FAT (g) | 1.0 |
| CARBS (g) | 9.0 |
| SUGAR (g) | 8.0 |
| FIBER (g) | 1.0 |
| PROTEIN (g) | 39.0 |
| SODIUM (g) | 2.82 |

**VARIATION**
If you don't like wasabi, replace it with 1 teaspoon of grated fresh ginger.

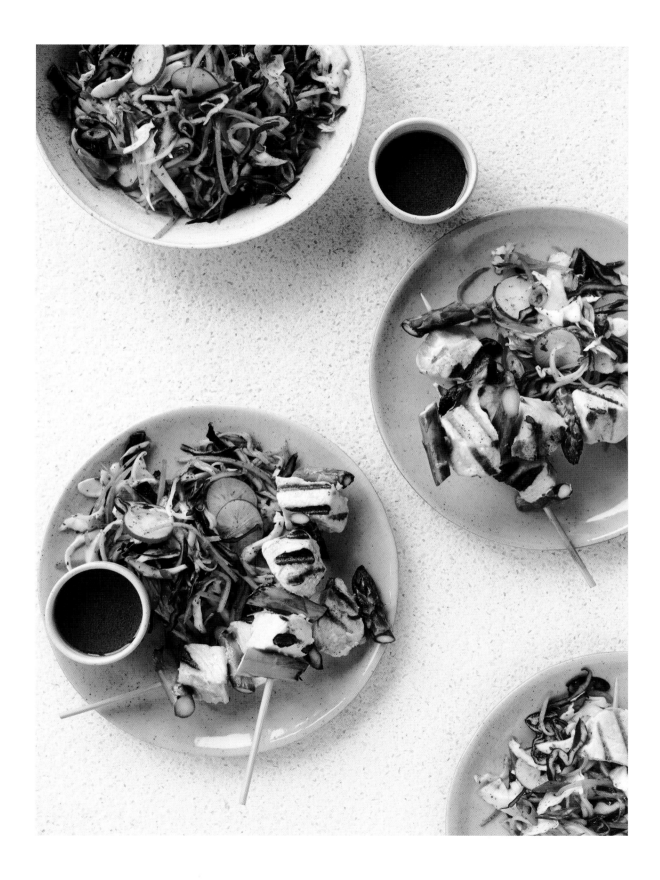

# ASIAN SLAW

**SERVES 4 AS A SIDE**

Green mangoes are unripe mangoes that are still hard to the touch. They are popular in cooking across Asia and are often used in salads, curries, rice dishes, pickles, and chutneys. Served raw and cut into strips, they add a tart flavor and welcome crunch to this crisp slaw. If you can't get ahold of unripe mangoes, use a couple of Granny Smith apples instead. Serve this with lean chicken, pork, or fish to make it more filling without adding many more calories.

½ small red cabbage, core removed and leaves finely shredded
½ small green cabbage, core removed and leaves finely shredded
2 carrots, grated
3½ ounces radishes, trimmed and sliced
2 spring onions, trimmed and thinly sliced
1 green mango, peeled and julienned
½ to 1 red chile, seeded and finely chopped (optional)

**FOR THE DRESSING**
½ small bunch of cilantro, chopped
½-inch piece of fresh ginger, minced
Juice of 3 limes
½ tablespoon fish sauce
½ teaspoon rice vinegar
2 teaspoons agave syrup

**1.** Put all the vegetables and the mango into a bowl with the chile, if using.

**2.** To make the dressing, put the cilantro and ginger into a blender and blitz until very finely chopped. Add the remaining dressing ingredients and blend until smooth. Taste and adjust the flavors as necessary.

**3.** Pour the dressing over the vegetables and mix really well before serving.

| PER SERVING | |
| --- | --- |
| CALORIES | 105 |
| FAT (g) | 1.0 |
| SATURATED FAT (g) | 0.1 |
| CARBS (g) | 18.0 |
| SUGAR (g) | 17.0 |
| FIBER (g) | 7.0 |
| PROTEIN (g) | 3.0 |
| SODIUM (g) | 0.47 |

# ONE-PAN CHICKEN WITH LIMA BEANS, LEEKS, AND SPINACH

**SERVES 4 TO 6**

Cooking everything together in one pan has some great advantages—all the prep work is done up front, so you can get on with other things once it's in the oven, the flavors really come together as they cook, and there is only one pan to wash up when you're finished. It makes for a great family-friendly recipe and no arguments about who's doing the dishes. Serve with roasted baby potatoes in their skins or the Sweet Potato Chips on page 241 if weight loss isn't a priority.

1 whole chicken, cut up, or 2 breasts,
  2 thighs, and 2 drumsticks, skin removed
Sea salt and freshly ground black pepper
1 tablespoon olive oil
1 head garlic, cut in half horizontally
1 leek, trimmed, halved lengthwise, and sliced
¾ cup dry white wine
1½ cups chicken or vegetable stock
2 thyme sprigs
2 (15-ounce) cans lima beans, drained and rinsed
8 ounces baby spinach leaves

**1.** Preheat the oven to 350°F. Season the chicken with salt and pepper.

**2.** Place a large roasting pan on the stovetop to heat up over medium-high heat and add the oil. Once hot, brown the chicken pieces on all sides until nicely colored. Turn the chicken skin side up.

**3.** Add the garlic to the pan, cut side down, then add the leek slices and stir around in the oil.

**4.** Pour in the white wine and allow to bubble for 2 minutes, then add the stock. Use a wooden spoon to scrape up any bits stuck to the bottom.

**5.** Turn off the heat and add the thyme sprigs, lima beans, and spinach, nestling them between the chicken pieces. Season with a pinch of salt and pepper and mix everything together, then put the pan into the oven. Bake for 35 to 40 minutes, until the chicken is cooked through. Give the contents of the pan a stir occasionally to make sure everything is cooking evenly.

**6.** Remove the pan from the oven and leave to rest for 5 minutes before serving in warm shallow bowls.

**TO MAKE IT LESS LEAN**
Leave the skin on the chicken if you aren't watching your weight, and follow the recipe above, but be careful not to pour the wine or stock over the browned skin because it won't crisp up properly in the oven.

| PER SERVING | |
| --- | --- |
| CALORIES | 509 |
| FAT (g) | 16.0 |
| SATURATED FAT (g) | 4.0 |
| CARBS (g) | 18.0 |
| SUGAR (g) | 2.0 |
| FIBER (g) | 10.0 |
| PROTEIN (g) | 58.0 |
| SODIUM (g) | 0.62 |

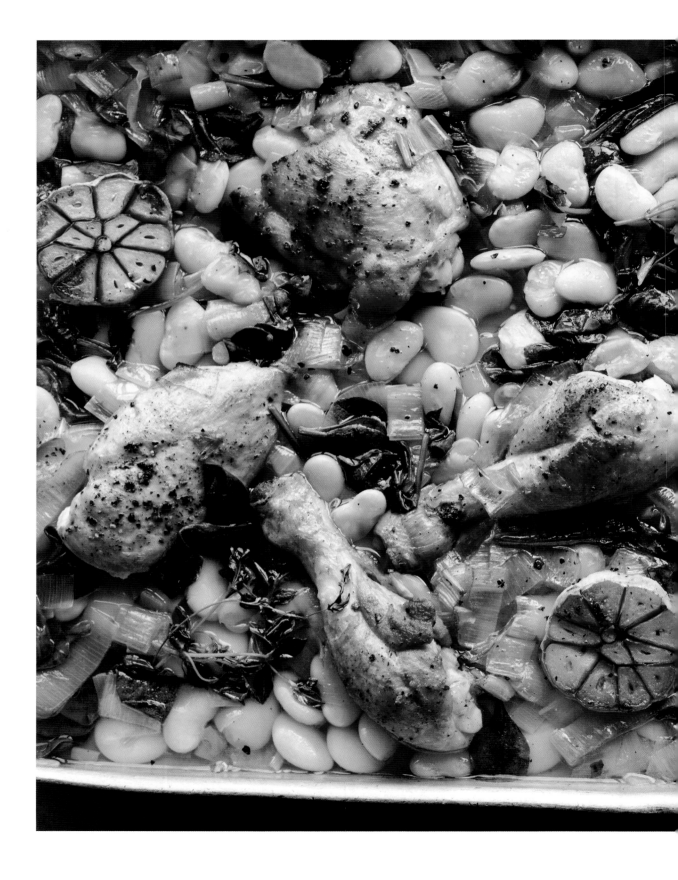

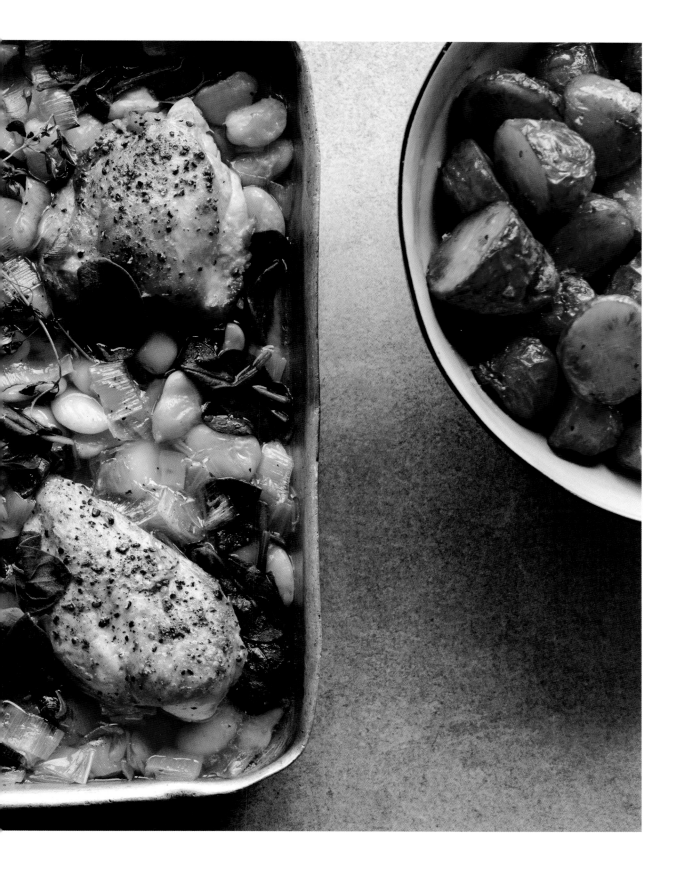

# DUCK BREAST WITH BRAISED FENNEL AND ORANGE GREMOLATA

**SERVES 4**

Duck has a reputation of being really fatty, but if you remove the skin, the breasts are actually leaner than steak and include more iron than a chicken breast. Braising fennel not only softens it, it also mellows the strong anise flavor of the raw vegetable while the orange gremolata adds zest and freshness. This is equally delicious served straight from the oven or at room temperature.

2 fennel bulbs
Olive oil
Sea salt and freshly ground black pepper
Juice of ½ orange (zest used below)
4 (5-ounce) duck breasts, skin removed
    and trimmed of fat

**FOR THE GREMOLATA**
Zest of 1 orange (from above)
½ small bunch of flat-leaf parsley, leaves
    finely chopped
1 garlic clove, peeled and very finely chopped
Sea salt and freshly ground black pepper

1. Preheat the oven to 350°F.

2. Remove any green fronds from the fennel and reserve for serving. Slice the fennel in half lengthwise, then slice each half in half again.

3. Heat a large casserole dish over medium heat. Add a dash of olive oil and brown the fennel pieces on each side until dark golden (you may have to do this in batches, depending on the size of your dish).

4. Arrange the browned fennel pieces in a single layer in the pan and season with a little salt and pepper. Squeeze over the orange juice and pour in ⅓ cup of water. Put the lid on and transfer to the oven.

5. Braise the fennel for 25 to 35 minutes, until very soft but still retaining its shape. Check the dish occasionally, and if the fennel looks like it is drying out, add another ⅓ cup of water.

6. Meanwhile, for the gremolata, mix together the orange zest, parsley, and garlic in a small bowl. Season with a little pinch of salt and pepper.

7. Place a large skillet over high heat and add a little oil. When it's hot, add the duck breasts. Cook for around 12 minutes for medium. Remove the meat from the pan and allow to rest for 5 minutes, then slice.

8. Once the fennel is cooked, remove from the oven and leave to rest for 5 minutes, then serve with the sliced duck breast and gremolata, with any reserved fronds sprinkled on top.

**GOOD TO KNOW**
So much of the goodness in citrus fruit is in the zest, which is very fiber- and nutrient-dense, so grate it over your food whenever you can. It livens up fish, chicken, pasta, salads, dips, cocktails . . .

| PER SERVING | |
| --- | --- |
| CALORIES | 352 |
| FAT (g) | 19.0 |
| SATURATED FAT (g) | 6.0 |
| CARBS (g) | 3.0 |
| SUGAR (g) | 3.0 |
| FIBER (g) | 4.0 |
| PROTEIN (g) | 39.0 |
| SODIUM (g) | 0.4 |

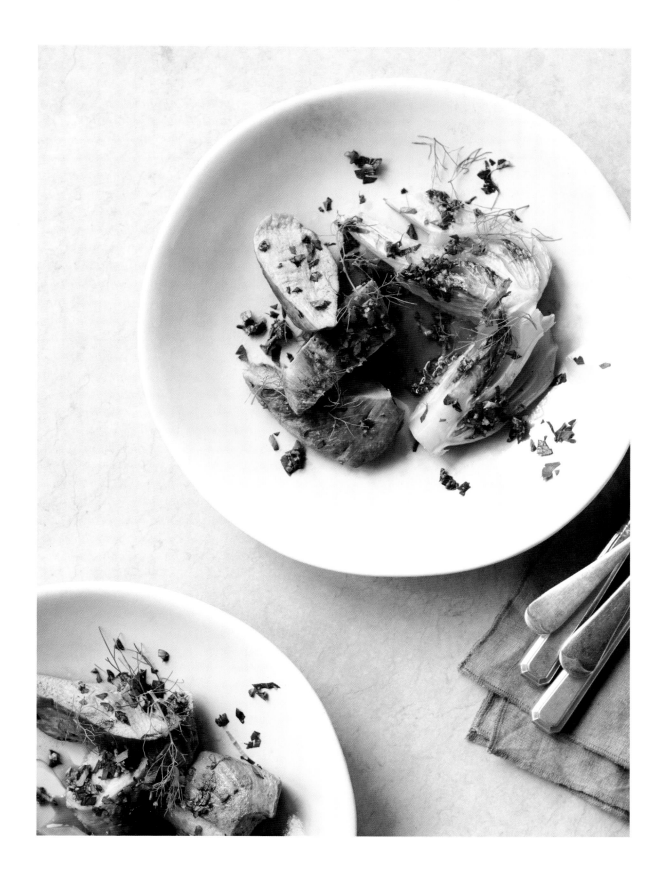

# VELVETED PORK LOIN WITH GINGER SUSHI RICE AND PICKLED VEGETABLES

**SERVES 2**

Velveting is a Chinese cooking method that keeps meat tender when it is exposed to high temperatures. By marinating the pork in a combination of cornstarch and egg white, you are literally creating a barrier that seals in the moisture that is usually lost in cooking. Velveting works particularly well with lean meats that are prone to drying out, such as chicken breasts and pork loin, but it also works brilliantly with strips of beef and duck.

1 egg white
2 tablespoons cornstarch
1½ tablespoons light soy sauce
1½ teaspoons honey
2 garlic cloves, peeled and finely chopped
2½-inch piece of fresh ginger, peeled
10½ ounces pork tenderloin, trimmed of sinew and cut into ¼-inch slices
3½ tablespoons rice vinegar
1 teaspoon sugar
1 teaspoon fine sea salt
½ medium cucumber, seeded, halved lengthwise, and sliced
1 red chile, seeded and thinly sliced
3 ounces radishes, trimmed and thinly sliced
1 cup sushi rice
Pea shoots, to serve

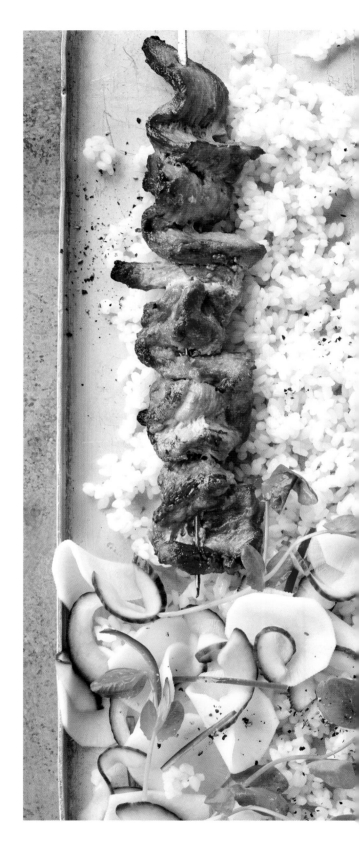

| PER SERVING | |
| --- | --- |
| CALORIES | 548 |
| FAT (g) | 4.0 |
| SATURATED FAT (g) | 1.0 |
| CARBS (g) | 84.0 |
| SUGAR (g) | 8.0 |
| FIBER (g) | 2.0 |
| PROTEIN (g) | 42.0 |
| SODIUM (g) | 3.07 |

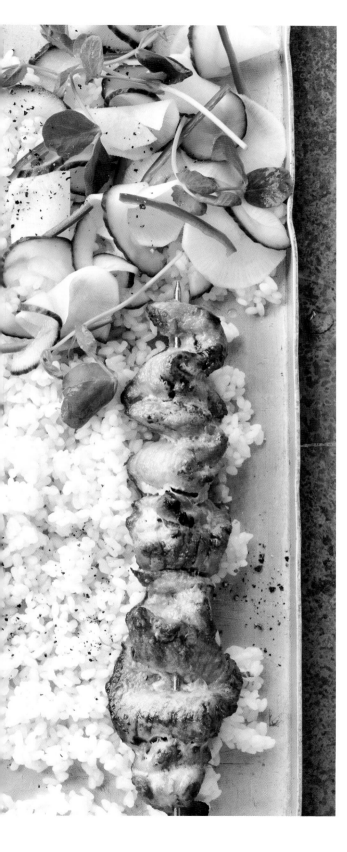

1. Whisk together the egg white, cornstarch, soy sauce, honey, and chopped garlic in a large bowl.

2. Grate the ginger into a sieve over a bowl, then use the back of a spoon to squeeze the juice from the ginger into the bowl. Mix the squeezed ginger flesh into the egg white mixture, then cover the ginger juice and store in the fridge until needed.

3. Put the pork slices into the egg white mixture and make sure they are all well covered. Cover and leave to marinate for a minimum of 2 hours, but preferably overnight.

4. When ready to cook, mix the reserved ginger juice with the rice vinegar, sugar, and salt. Tip all but 2 tablespoons of the liquid into a bowl, then add the cucumber, chile, and radishes and toss them in the liquid. Leave the vegetables to steep for 1 hour, stirring occasionally.

5. Soak the sushi rice in cold water for 20 minutes, then strain through a sieve and rinse under cold water. Tip the rice into a small saucepan and add 1 cup of water. Bring the water to a boil over high heat, then cover with a tight lid, reduce the heat to its lowest setting, and cook for 13 minutes—do not remove the lid at any point.

6. After 13 minutes, turn the heat off and leave the rice to stand for a minimum of 5 minutes without removing the lid.

7. Preheat the broiler to high.

8. Thread the marinated meat onto two skewers (if using bamboo skewers, soak them in water for 20 minutes beforehand). Broil for 8 minutes on one side, then flip and cook for an additional 4 minutes on the second side, or until nicely browned and cooked through.

9. When ready to serve, remove the lid from the rice pan and pour in the remaining 2 tablespoons of ginger juice mixture. Use a fork to rough up the rice and to help it absorb the liquid.

10. Drain the pickled vegetables and serve them with the rice, pork skewers, and a handful of pea shoots.

# VENISON CARPACCIO WITH CELERIAC SLAW

**SERVES 4**

Venison is naturally very lean and has more protein than any other red meat, making it very filling—excellent for satisfying the appetite when you are watching what you eat. It should always be served pink in the middle, but I also love it very rare like this, as it's meltingly tender and full of flavor. An autumnal salad with a yogurt-based dressing like this one is the perfect garnish.

1 venison fillet (approximately 1 pound)
2 tablespoons canola oil
Sea salt and freshly ground black pepper
1½ tablespoons cider vinegar
1½ teaspoons Dijon mustard
¼ cup 0% fat Greek yogurt
1 small celeriac, peeled and julienned
1 Granny Smith apple, peeled,
   cored, and julienned
⅓ cup walnut pieces
¼ cup raisins
3 celery stalks, trimmed and thickly
   sliced diagonally

**TO SERVE**
Watercress
⅓ cup blackberries, halved

1. Place a large skillet over high heat. Brush the venison all over with a little of the canola oil, then season with salt and pepper.

2. When the pan is smoking hot, quickly brown the venison all over. Remove the meat from the pan and leave to cool to room temperature.

3. Lay a piece of plastic wrap on a board and place the venison on top. Roll the venison in the plastic until you have a tight sausage shape and secure it tightly at each end. Put the venison into the fridge and leave to sit for 2 hours, or preferably overnight.

4. Just before serving, whisk together the remaining oil, the cider vinegar, mustard, and yogurt with ¼ cup of warm water.

5. Place the julienned celeriac, apple, walnut pieces, raisins, and celery in a bowl, pour over the dressing, then toss until everything is well coated.

6. Unravel the venison from the plastic wrap and slice it as thinly as you can. Divide the slices among four plates, laying them flat in a single layer. Top with the celeriac salad and finish with a big handful of watercress and a few blackberry halves scattered over the top.

| PER SERVING | |
| --- | --- |
| CALORIES | 333 |
| FAT (g) | 17.0 |
| SATURATED FAT (g) | 2.0 |
| CARBS (g) | 11.0 |
| SUGAR (g) | 11.0 |
| FIBER (g) | 4.0 |
| PROTEIN (g) | 32.0 |
| SODIUM (g) | 0.51 |

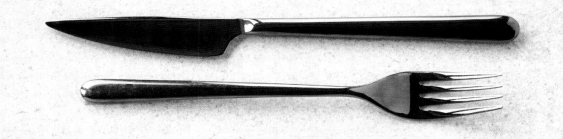
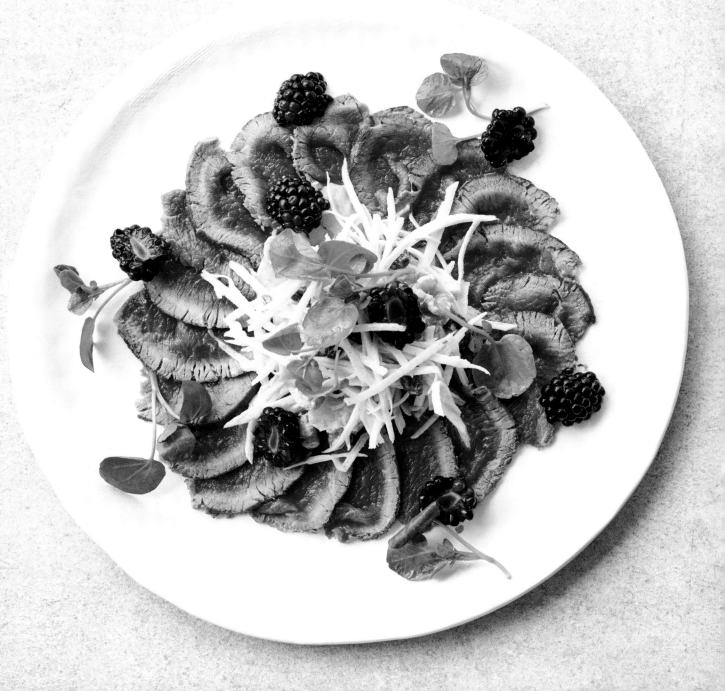

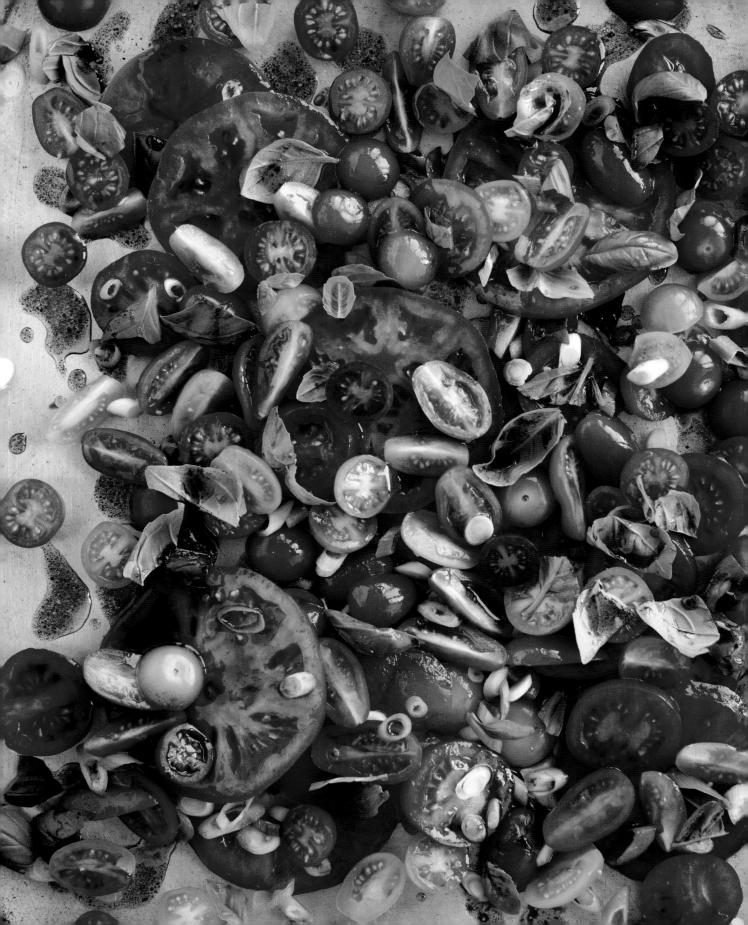

# MARINATED TOMATO SALAD

**SERVES 4 AS A SIDE**

Marinating tomatoes for a couple of hours before you eat them totally transforms a regular tomato salad into a sensational one. Trust me, it's worth doing. The flavors really intensify, as does the nutrient content, and the tomatoes come alive. Choose ripe tomatoes of different colors and sizes, and use a high quality extra virgin olive oil—it will make all the difference.

2¼ pounds ripe tomatoes
3 spring onions, or 1 small shallot,
   very finely diced
Small bunch of basil, leaves only
1½ tablespoons balsamic or sherry vinegar
¼ cup extra virgin olive oil
Sea salt and freshly ground black pepper

**1.** Slice, halve, or quarter the tomatoes, depending on their size, and put them all into a large serving bowl.

**2.** Sprinkle over the diced spring onions or shallot, then tear the basil leaves and add them on top.

**3.** Pour in the vinegar and olive oil and add a good pinch of salt and pepper, then, using your hands, gently mix these through the tomatoes, taking care not to bruise any of the ripe fruit.

**4.** Cover the dish and leave at room temperature for at least 1 hour or up to 3 hours before serving.

| PER SERVING | |
| --- | --- |
| CALORIES | 149 |
| FAT (g) | 11.0 |
| SATURATED FAT (g) | 2.0 |
| CARBS (g) | 9.0 |
| SUGAR (g) | 8.0 |
| FIBER (g) | 3.0 |
| PROTEIN (g) | 2.0 |
| SODIUM (g) | 0.02 |

# GUILT-FREE TREATS

# ICED GREEN TEA

**SERVES 4**

In health-conscious California, green tea—with all its antioxidants, flavonoids, and polyphenols (phytochemicals valued for their protective properties)—is even more popular than black tea. Make a big pitcher of it and sip it through the day to keep you hydrated and take your mind off sugary snacks at the same time.

4 green tea bags
Runny honey, to taste
1 unwaxed lemon, sliced

**1.** Put the tea bags into a heatproof container such as a large teapot or pitcher. Pour over 5 cups of just-boiled water and sweeten with runny honey (1 to 1½ tablespoons) to taste.

**2.** Add the lemon slices and leave to steep until cooled, then remove the tea bags.

**3.** Taste and add more honey if necessary.

**4.** Serve in tall glasses with lots of ice.

| PER SERVING | |
| --- | --- |
| CALORIES | 23 |
| FAT (g) | 0.1 |
| SATURATED FAT (g) | 0.0 |
| CARBS (g) | 5.0 |
| SUGAR (g) | 4.0 |
| FIBER (g) | 0.5 |
| PROTEIN (g) | 1.0 |
| SODIUM (g) | 0.01 |

**VARIATIONS**
You can add different flavors to this tea—slices of fresh ginger or lime are brilliant to add during the steeping process, as are sprigs of herbs such as mint or lemon thyme, or even metabolism-boosting spices like cayenne.

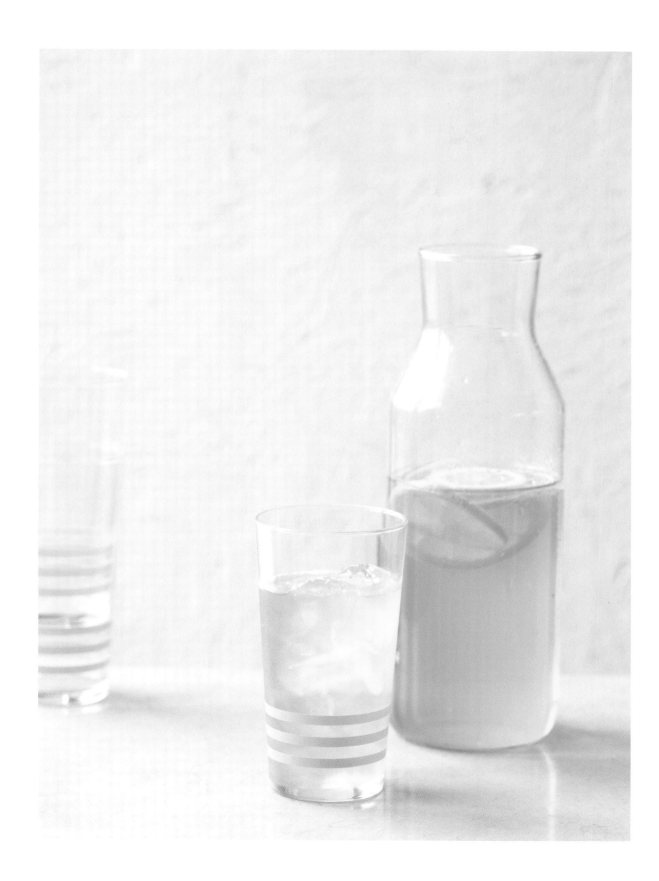

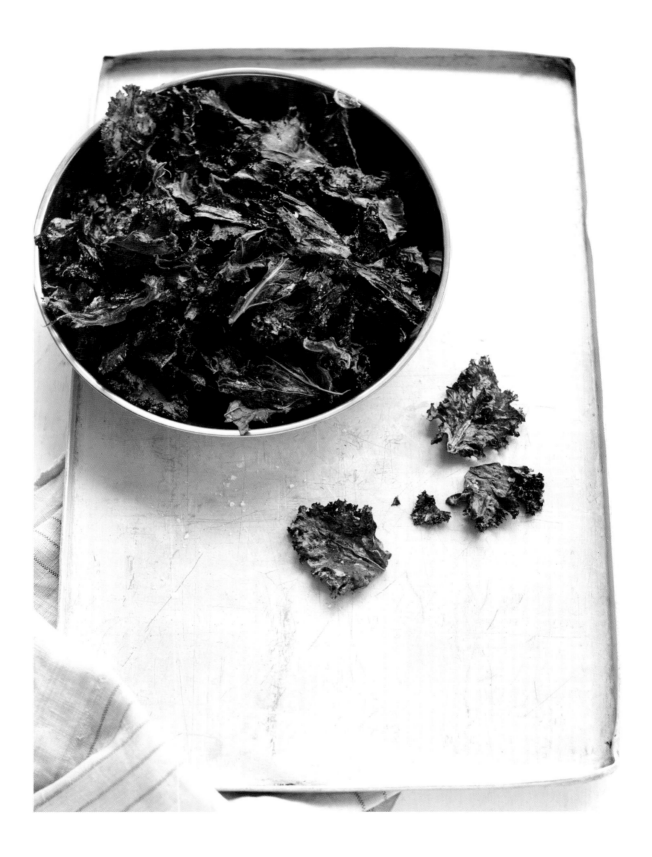

# MAPLE SOY KALE CHIPS
**SERVES 4**

Roasting kale in this way changes it from a raw cabbage leaf into a crisp snack that tastes like the crispy seaweed you get in Chinese restaurants but is much better for you. Kale chips are also delicious crumbled over salads or sprinkled over Asian dishes, giving them an intense, salty hit.

1 bunch of kale, stems removed, leaves washed and dried
1 tablespoon maple syrup
1 tablespoon olive oil
1 teaspoon soy sauce
Pinch of salt

1. Preheat the oven to 300°F.

2. Slice the kale into bite-size pieces the same size as potato chips.

3. Put the maple syrup, olive oil, soy sauce, and salt into a large bowl and mix together. Add the kale to the bowl and massage the marinade into the leaves, making sure that every piece of kale is coated.

4. Spread the kale in a single layer on one or two baking sheets. Put the sheets into the oven and bake for 7 to 10 minutes. After 5 minutes, check the kale and swap the shelves if using more than one sheet. Continue to bake until the kale is crisp but not burning. Some pieces may cook faster than others, in which case remove the pieces that are crisp and continue to bake the remaining pieces until they are also crisp. Leave to cool.

5. Once cooled, they can be stored in an airtight container for up to a week.

**VARIATIONS**
Kale chips are a great vehicle for lots of different flavors, such as chile, lime, wasabi, or Parmesan cheese. For paprika chips, follow the method above, but marinate the kale in 1 tablespoon olive oil, 1 teaspoon smoked paprika, ½ teaspoon garlic granules, 1 teaspoon chile flakes (optional), and a pinch of salt.

| PER SERVING | |
| --- | --- |
| CALORIES | 59 |
| FAT (g) | 4.0 |
| SATURATED FAT (g) | 1.0 |
| CARBS (g) | 4.0 |
| SUGAR (g) | 4.0 |
| FIBER (g) | 2.0 |
| PROTEIN (g) | 2.0 |
| SODIUM (g) | 0.23 |

# SMOKY SPICED POPCORN

**SERVES 4**

Making your own popcorn is really easy and, if you keep the amount of oil down, much better for you than commercial brands, which can be just as fattening as potato chips. Spicing up your popcorn is a clever way to help you eat less of it, too. This combination of sweet, smoky paprika and warming garam masala is amazing, but you could also experiment with other favorite spices like cinnamon, cumin, or black pepper.

2 tablespoons sunflower oil
⅓ cup popcorn kernels
Pinch of salt
1 teaspoon sweet smoked paprika
½ teaspoon garam masala

1. Place a large saucepan with a tight-fitting lid over medium-high heat and add the oil.

2 When the oil is very hot (see below), sprinkle in the popcorn kernels and put the lid on. Once you hear the kernels start to pop, give the pan a little shake approximately every 30 seconds. When the sound of the corn popping has died down, turn off the heat and carefully remove the lid.

3. Put the salt, paprika, and garam masala into a small bowl and mix together until thoroughly blended.

4. Tip the popcorn into a large baking sheet and sprinkle with the spiced salt, tossing gently until coated evenly. Eat immediately, or keep in an airtight container for a couple of days.

| PER SERVING | |
| --- | --- |
| CALORIES | 141 |
| FAT (g) | 7.0 |
| SATURATED FAT (g) | 1.0 |
| CARBS (g) | 15.0 |
| SUGAR (g) | 0.3 |
| FIBER (g) | 3.0 |
| PROTEIN (g) | 3.0 |
| SODIUM (g) | 0.37 |

**HOW TO MAKE POPCORN**
A clever way of telling when the oil is hot enough before adding the popcorn is to add three kernels first. When all three of them have popped, the oil is ready to go.

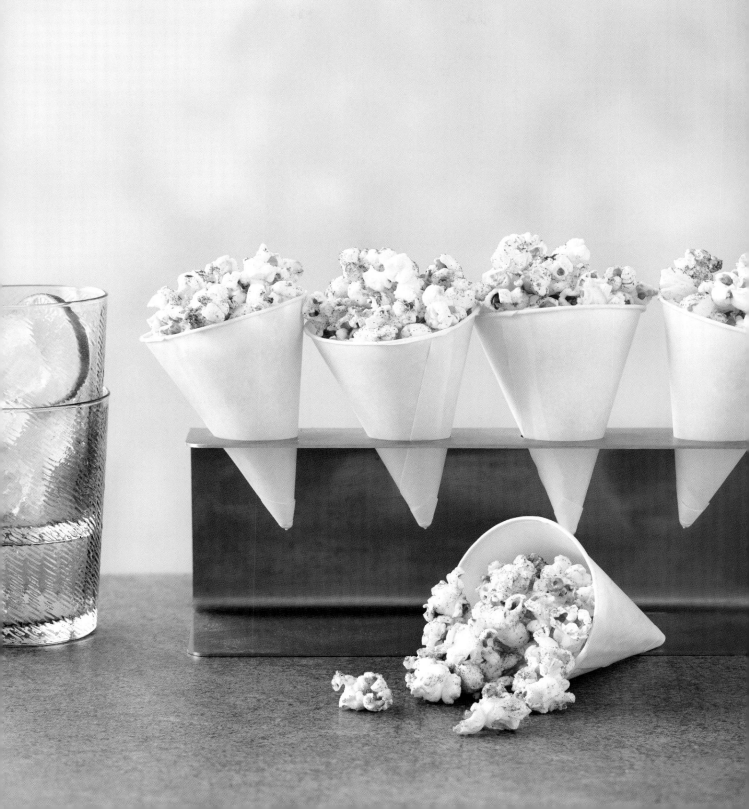

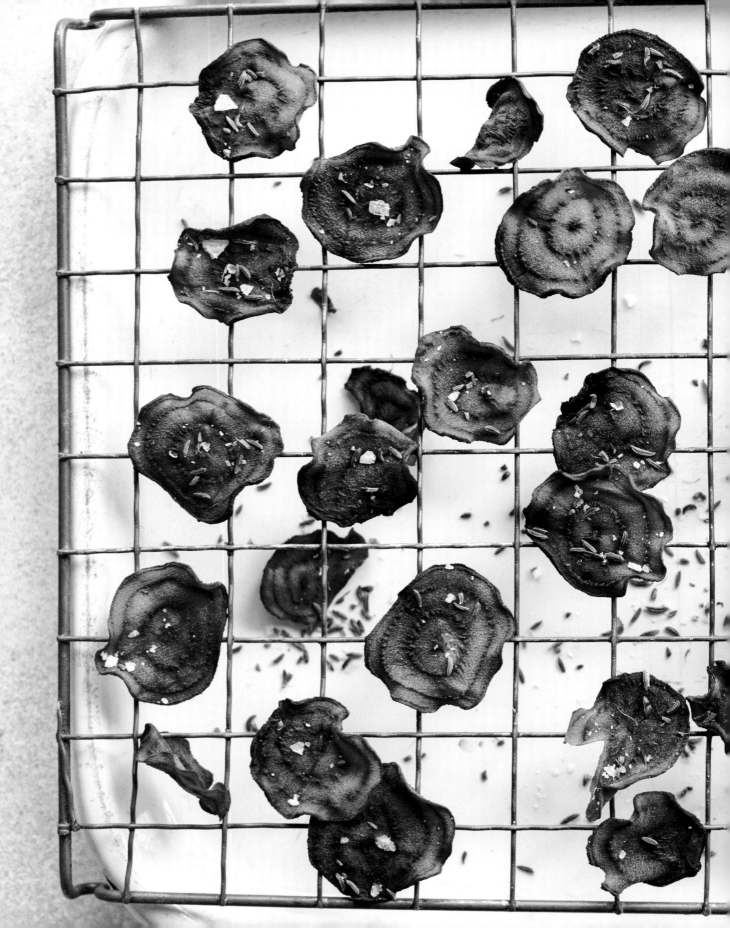

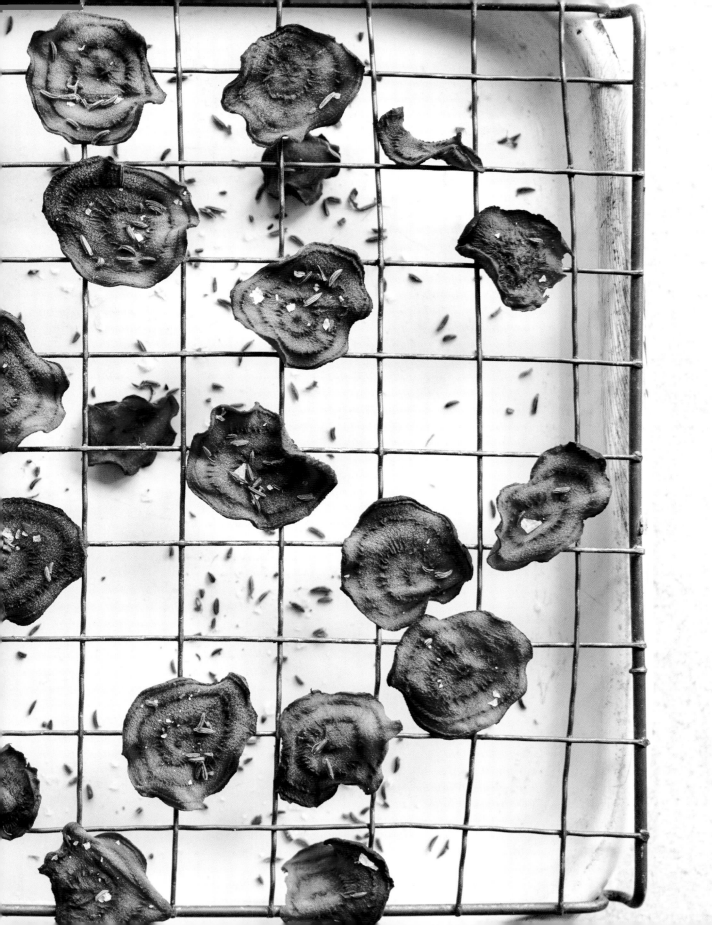

# CARAWAY BEET CHIPS

**SERVES 4**

Traditional chips are off the menu when trying to lose weight because they are so high in fat and because we tend to eat more than we should once we start, but these healthy beet chips are fat- and guilt-free, so you can eat as many as you like and they make a contribution to your daily veggie goals. They go brilliantly with dips like Baba Ghanoush (page 95) and Hummus (page 94). If you don't eat them all in one sitting, the chips will keep in an airtight container for up to two days.

3 medium beets (approximately 12 ounces), peeled
2 teaspoons caraway seeds, toasted
1 teaspoon sea salt

1. Preheat the oven to 325°F.

2. Place two cooling racks on top of two baking sheets. If you don't have cooling racks, use baking sheets lined with waxed paper. (This will take longer, so don't remove the beets from the oven until they are definitely crisp.)

3. Thinly slice the beets, ideally with a mandoline or a very sharp knife.

4. Lay the slices out in a thin layer on the racks, trying not to let them overlap. Bake the slices in the oven for 15 to 20 minutes.

5. Meanwhile, crush the toasted caraway seeds and sea salt together in a mortar and pestle.

6. After 15 minutes, check the chips, and if they're not quite crisp, continue to bake—the time will depend on how thick the beet slices are.

7. When the chips have finished baking, remove the sheets from the oven and leave them to cool on the racks.

8. When cooled, transfer the chips to a bowl and sprinkle with the caraway salt, carefully tossing them to ensure an even coating.

| PER SERVING | |
| --- | --- |
| CALORIES | 38 |
| FAT (g) | 0.3 |
| SATURATED FAT (g) | 0.0 |
| CARBS (g) | 6.0 |
| SUGAR (g) | 5.0 |
| FIBER (g) | 2.0 |
| PROTEIN (g) | 2.0 |
| SODIUM (g) | 1.36 |

# SPICED APPLE SORBET

**SERVES 4**

Sorbet is much lighter than ice cream in terms of fat content, but it's still packed with flavor, which makes this the perfect sweet hit for the end of a meal, particularly in autumn when apples are at their best. By choosing red apples the sorbet will have a hint of pink from the skins, which makes it very pretty as well as refreshing—a perfect palate cleanser.

6 medium red apples,
  quartered and cored
1 tablespoon maple syrup
Juice of 1 lemon
2 teaspoons ground cinnamon
½ teaspoon ground cardamom
1 teaspoon ground ginger

1. Chop the apples into chunks and put them into a saucepan with the maple syrup, 1 cup of water, the lemon juice, cinnamon, cardamom, and ginger. Bring to a simmer over medium-low heat, stirring often, and cook until the apples have completely collapsed and an apple purée has formed.

2. Taste the mixture and add a little more maple syrup if needed, remembering that when the mixture is frozen the flavors will be dulled slightly, so any sweetness or sourness will not be so pronounced.

3. Pour into a food processor and process until completely smooth.

4. Put the mixture into a freezer-safe container with a lid and freeze for at least 6 hours, until set.

5. Remove the sorbet from the freezer 15 minutes before serving to soften slightly.

| PER SERVING | |
| --- | --- |
| CALORIES | 98 |
| FAT (g) | 1.0 |
| SATURATED FAT (g) | 0.2 |
| CARBS (g) | 20.0 |
| SUGAR (g) | 20.0 |
| FIBER (g) | 3.0 |
| PROTEIN (g) | 1.0 |
| SODIUM (g) | 0.01 |

# BANANA "ICE CREAM"

**SERVES 4**

My daughter Tilly introduced me to this genius recipe . . . it's a one-ingredient, dairy-free, fat-free ice cream with no added sugar that you don't need an ice cream machine to make—it's incredible! You can add all sorts of things to the base recipe, like peanut butter, frozen berries, chocolate chips, cocoa nibs, coconut flakes, or chopped nuts (see page 277 for a coconut and chocolate version). Just make sure you don't add any liquid or it will lose its ice cream–like consistency.

4 ripe bananas, peeled

1. Slice the bananas into chunks and put them into a freezer container. Put the container into the freezer and leave overnight or until frozen solid.

2. When ready to make the ice cream, put the frozen banana pieces into a food processor and pulse to break them up into small pieces. Scrape down the sides of the food processor, then blend until the banana is smooth and creamy, stopping regularly to scrape down the sides.

3. Eat immediately for a soft-serve consistency or put it back into a freezer-proof container and freeze for 1 hour, or until hard.

| PER SERVING | |
|---|---|
| CALORIES | 86 |
| FAT (g) | 0.1 |
| SATURATED FAT (g) | 0.0 |
| CARBS (g) | 19.0 |
| SUGAR (g) | 17.0 |
| FIBER (g) | 1.0 |
| PROTEIN (g) | 1.0 |
| SODIUM (g) | 0.04 |

# COCONUT ICE POPS

**MAKES 6 ICE POPS**

This is another excellent dairy-free ice cream that doesn't need an ice cream machine. You can make it without the fruit, as the coconut has such a delicious flavor on its own, or stir through some desiccated coconut and lime zest for extra texture and bite. This is the kind of guilt-free indulgence that really helps to keep you on track when willpower is beginning to weaken.

1 cup coconut milk
1 tablespoon maple syrup
3½ ounces fresh or frozen fruit, such as blueberries, raspberries, or mango chunks

1. Put the coconut milk and maple syrup into a pitcher and mix until completely combined. Stir in the fruit.

2. Divide the mixture among the ice pop molds.

3. Put ice pop sticks into the molds and transfer to the freezer for at least 4 hours but ideally overnight.

4. To serve, remove from the freezer and allow to warm slightly before pulling the ice pops out of the molds.

**VARIATIONS**
These are great made with blueberries, raspberries, blackberries, or mango, all of which freeze really well. Keep bags of frozen fruits in the freezer so you can make these ice pops all year round even if your fruit bowl is empty.

| PER SERVING | |
| --- | --- |
| CALORIES | 71 |
| FAT (g) | 6.0 |
| SATURATED FAT (g) | 5.0 |
| CARBS (g) | 4.0 |
| SUGAR (g) | 3.0 |
| FIBER (g) | 1.0 |
| PROTEIN (g) | 1.0 |
| SODIUM (g) | 0.01 |

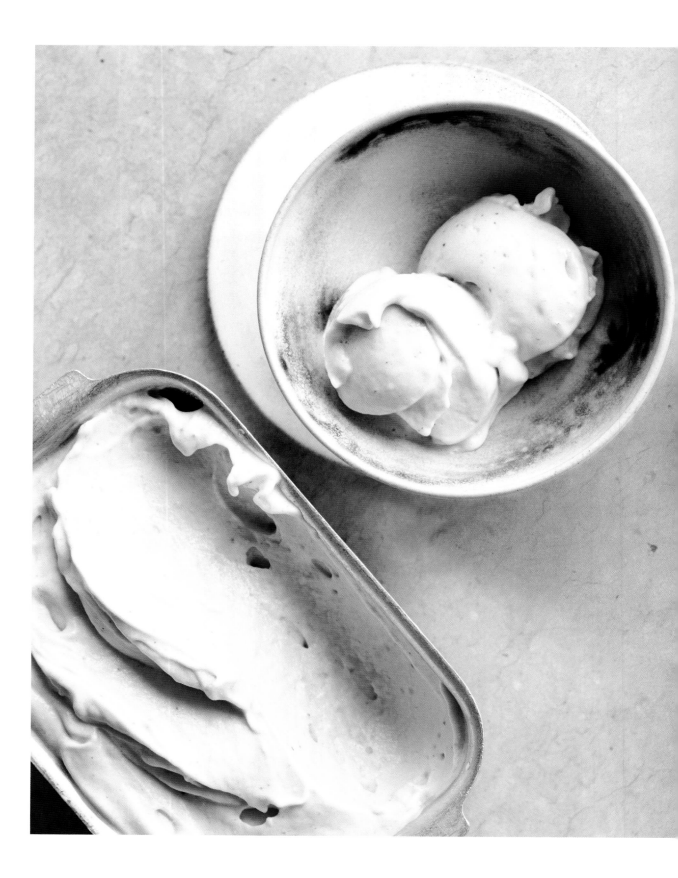

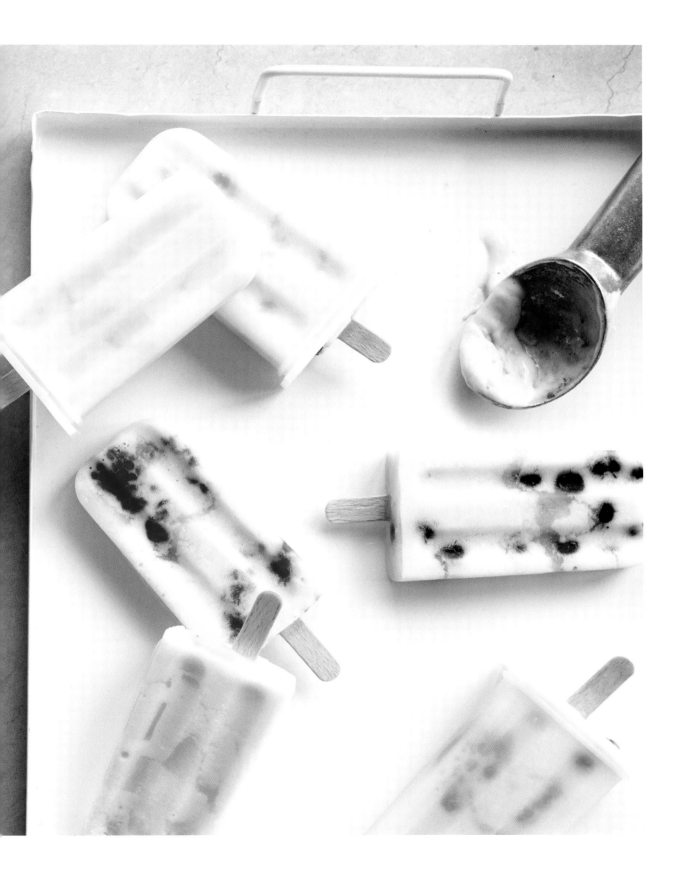

# CARROT CAKE MACAROONS
**MAKES 18 MACAROONS**

These macaroons are not to be muddled up with French macarons, which are those delicate meringue spaceships that are full of sugar and can be a bit tricky to cook outside a professional pastry kitchen. These are the coconut macaroons of my childhood, updated to taste a lot like carrot cake but without all that frosting. When cake is off the menu, have a couple of these to keep the sweet cravings at bay.

2½ cups unsweetened desiccated coconut
1½ teaspoons ground cinnamon
1 teaspoon ground ginger
½ teaspoon freshly grated nutmeg
½ cup chopped walnuts
1 large carrot, grated
½ cup coconut sugar
4 egg whites
Pinch of salt

1. Preheat the oven to 350°F.

2. Put the coconut, cinnamon, ginger, and nutmeg into a bowl and mix well.

3. Add the chopped walnuts, grated carrot, coconut sugar, egg whites, and a pinch of salt and mix together until everything is fully incorporated.

4. Line a baking sheet with parchment paper and, using a 2-tablespoon cookie scoop, lightly pack in the mixture and then drop it onto the sheet, leaving a gap of about 1½ inches between them. If you don't have a cookie scoop, use your hands to shape into mounds that are roughly circular.

5. Put the sheet into the oven and bake for 15 to 20 minutes, until lightly browned and firm on the outside. Leave to cool on a wire rack before serving.

| PER MACAROON | |
| --- | --- |
| CALORIES | 120 |
| FAT (g) | 10.0 |
| SATURATED FAT (g) | 7.0 |
| CARBS (g) | 8.0 |
| SUGAR (g) | 5.0 |
| FIBER (g) | 2.0 |
| PROTEIN (g) | 2.0 |
| SODIUM (g) | .035 |

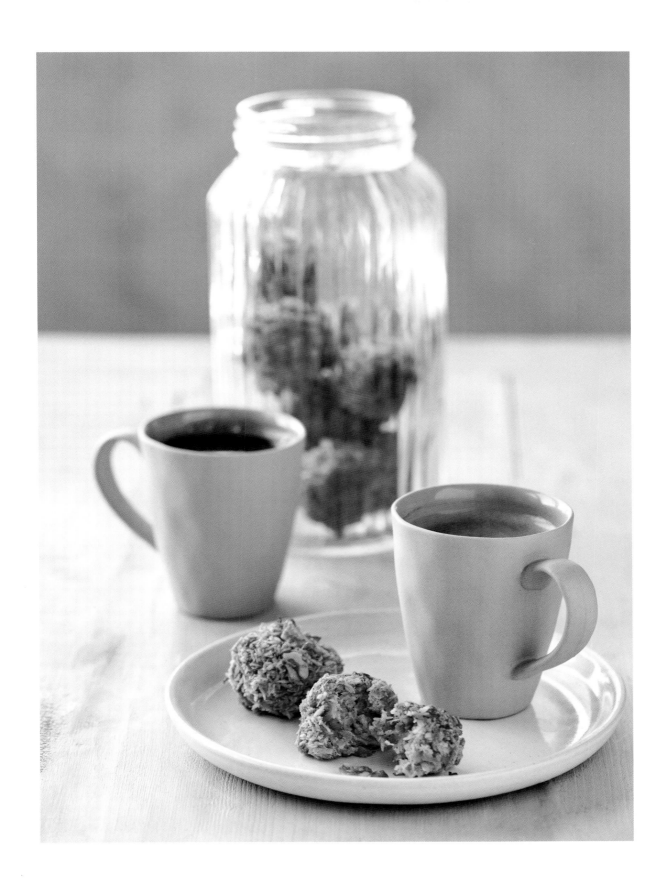

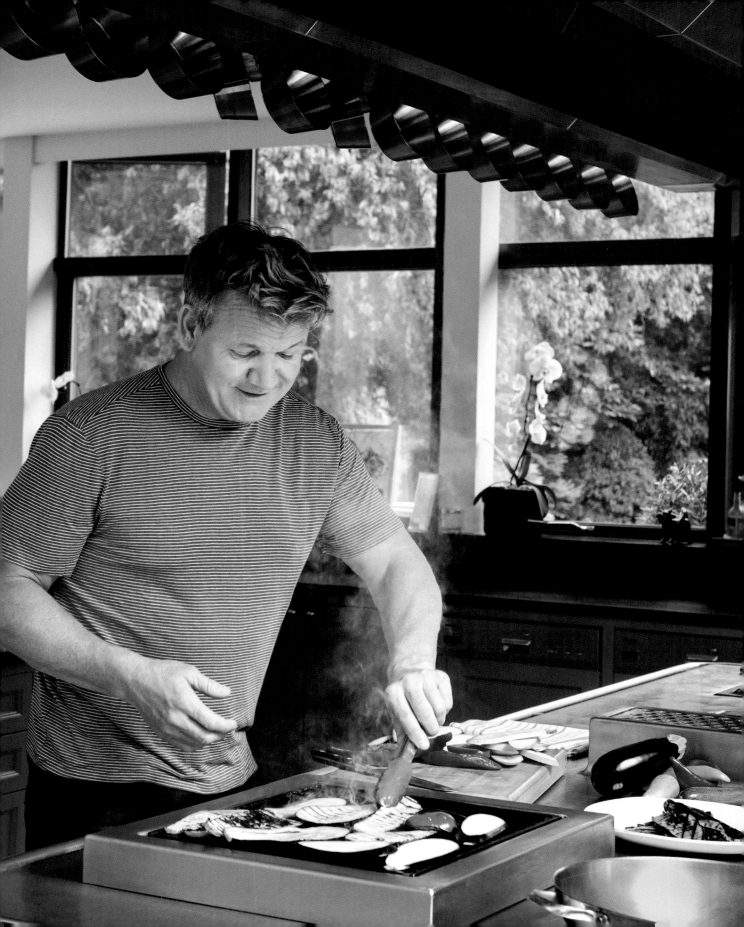

BOOSTING BREAKFASTS

LUNCHES FOR ACTIVE DAYS

CARB-LOADING
FOR THE NIGHT BEFORE

HIGH-PROTEIN RECOVERY
MEALS FOR THE EVENING AFTER

HIGH-ENERGY SNACKS
AND WELL-DESERVED TREATS

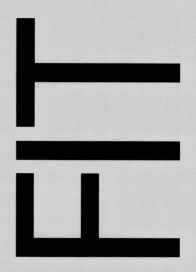

# EXERCISING IS COMPLETELY ESSENTIAL FOR MY WELL-BEING

Wherever I am in the world, I find a way to fit in a workout, run, or swim, often as soon as I arrive in a new city. It is my release from a very busy schedule and it helps me deal with the pressures I face. To keep myself fit and motivated, I always sign up for two major races a year; and when I'm not injured, I try to train properly at least three times a week, usually first thing in the morning, then I go for a huge bike ride on Sundays, sometimes with Tana or my son, Jack. So far, I have run fifteen marathons, three ultramarathons, four half Ironmans (a triathlon followed by a half marathon), and the world's toughest Ironman in Hawaii. And it's not just me—Tana has run seven marathons and two half Ironmans, too, and my daughter Megan recently competed in her first marathon at just eighteen!

Given that I am almost always in training for something, I have to keep an eye on the food I consume. Happily, my eating habits as a chef are quite similar to those recommended for athletes and sportsmen—eating little and often, which stabilizes blood sugar and keeps energy levels topped off, and not overeating, which slows the body down. When I'm training, I have to spend more time trying to get the right balance of carbohydrates, proteins, and fats needed for endurance. Fuel is just so important for performance—it not only helps you operate to the best of your abilities, it also reduces the risk of illness and injury and aids post-exercise recovery. If you aren't eating the right foods or getting enough liquids to keep you hydrated, you will struggle with fatigue or weakness and may even pick up strains and sprains.

Though each sport and each individual sportsman or sportswoman requires a slightly different combination of macronutrients to deliver the best results, there are a few general rules involving what to eat and when to eat it that apply to everyone. To put it simply, it's really important to get enough carbohydrates before you do any exercise, and equally important to follow up a tough session with some lean protein for muscle repair and some more carbs to restock your energy levels. It's also essential that you

drink enough water—becoming dehydrated will not only hinder your performance, it can be seriously bad for your health.

Understanding a bit more about basic sports nutrition and how the body works will help you prepare yourself for exercise challenges and maybe even improve your personal best! In this section, you will find recipes that have been designed to help you get the right balance of macronutrients when you need them and, given that they are some of my personal training favorites, they taste really good, too. The recipes here are sometimes higher in calories than in the previous two sections because they assume a very active lifestyle. And by active, I don't mean a water aerobics class once a week! This is food for training and endurance sessions that last at least an hour and much longer.

## CARB-LOADING

One of the key components of eating right for sports and training is the increased intake of carbohydrates before a big game or race. This is known as carb-loading and it is essential for fueling your muscles so they can deliver on the day. But how does it work? Putting it simply, when you eat carbs, they are broken down by the body to form glucose, which provides readily available energy for the body to use. Any extra glucose is stored in the muscles and liver in the form of glycogen for when the body needs it. Basically, glycogen is the reserve fuel that drives your muscles.

Because the body can store only a certain amount of glycogen at a time, it's important to keep topping the levels off, particularly before exercise. If you don't, you will tire easily, lack power, and underperform. Normally, carbohydrates should make up about a third of every meal, but this amount needs to increase as your exercise levels increase. And during the day or two before and on the morning of a big event, carb intake should rise to more than three-quarters of your food consumption.

Typically, the best carbohydrates to choose for exercise are the complex, unrefined varieties, which take longer for the body to break down and therefore release their energy more slowly. Good choices include whole-wheat bread, oatmeal, whole-wheat or brown rice pasta, noodles, brown rice, whole-wheat couscous, potatoes, parsnips, corn, peas, sweet potatoes, lentils, beans, and fruit. As you get closer to race day, however, you can eat more refined carbs like white rice, white pasta, bagels, and white bread, because they are so easy to digest and will lay down plenty of energy for physical exertion. It can feel quite repetitive and dull to eat pasta every night, so I make sure I vary the carbs I eat and serve them with punchy sauces and strong flavors to keep it interesting. (See page 227 for a list of chef's recipes for carb-loading.)

Most people start carb-loading a few days before a big race, but I like to start increasing my carb intake about six weeks in advance. It helps you to work out which carbs suit you in larger quantities and which ones don't, and it gets your body used to the increased carb levels. And with the increased glycogen levels, your training will be much more effective, too. Then, three or four days before the race, you should increase your intake further until it is making up 85 to 90 percent of your plate. Choose meals from the carb-loading chapter in this section for the eve of a race or event, then have a carb-rich breakfast early in the morning of the big day to further maximize your glycogen levels. For a final top-off, you should have an energy-charged snack at least thirty minutes before the start—less than thirty minutes and your body will still be digesting it when the starting gun sounds. Carb-loading in this way will ensure that you have the energy you need to get through the trial ahead, and I can't stress enough how important it is to get it right. Not having enough fuel in the tank can lead to low blood sugar, dizziness, and extreme exhaustion, otherwise known as "hitting the wall," and you will find yourself crashing out of the race.

**RECOVERY**

When it's all over and you are exhausted, elated, and aching all over, it is vital to eat or drink some form of protein, ideally within thirty minutes of finishing. Protein is needed for the repair and growth of muscles and, given that you have just put yours under incredible stress, they will need some TLC. Getting some protein in quickly will keep your muscles from being too sore (though they will still ache!) and help you to recover more quickly.

To maximize the efficiency of the protein, it's important to keep the amount of fat down because it can slow the uptake of the protein when you need it quickly. Therefore, choose lean sources like eggs, dairy products, and lean meat. A milk shake is ideal because not only does it supply protein and carbs, it also rehydrates the body at the same time and is easy to get your head around right after exercising, when you might not fancy a chicken sandwich. You need to keep eating protein for twenty-four hours after a big race, so pick one of the high-protein meals in the recovery section for your celebration feast—just make sure you get someone else to cook it while you have a well-deserved rest!

You also need yet more carbohydrates after exercise to refuel the glycogen levels in your muscles and again, at this point, it's okay to have fast-acting simple carbs that can be digested quickly and easily. You need to drink plenty of fluid, too, to replace all the liquid lost through sweat and to avoid dehydration. And then rest . . . most muscle repair happens while you are sleeping, so go to bed early and let your body do all the hard work.

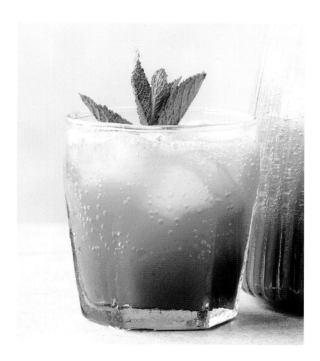

## HYDRATION FOR SPORTS

Drinking plenty of liquid is essential for good health but even more important when you are training and pushing yourself physically. Becoming dehydrated can seriously affect your performance, so make sure you take in plenty of liquid in advance. About two hours before a race, drink approximately 2 cups of water, diluted fruit juice, or a sports drink, and drink another ½ cup of fluid thirty minutes before you start. This should allow your body to get rid of any liquid it doesn't need before you get going. Drink small amounts while running to keep levels topped off as you sweat, and make sure you drink plenty of fluid afterward to get back to normal hydration levels. Also, be aware that different climates, seasons, altitudes, and weather can affect how much water you need, so do some research in advance and be prepared. Getting enough liquid for your body's needs will make all the difference on the day.

## ACTIVE KIDS

My four children are all really sporty. As I mentioned, my oldest daughter, Megan, has just run her first marathon at age eighteen and it can be hard to keep track of the different sports the rest of them play—water polo, netball, lacrosse, hockey, athletics, et cetera. They're all really keen on running, cycling, and swimming, too, and though I'm not sure whether it's genetic or purely driven by Tana and me, you would definitely say we're a pretty active family.

Getting the right nutrition matters even more for active kids and teenagers because they haven't finished growing yet. It is vital that they get enough energy from the food they eat to fuel activity, and a wide variety of micronutrients to keep them healthy. Make sure you provide carb-based meals for supper and breakfast on game days and have plenty of energy-boosting snacks like granola bars or Fig Bars (page 274) available for when they're needed. As with adults, protein is essential for muscle recovery, so encourage your kids to eat snacks like cheese, yogurt, or peanut butter sandwiches when it's all over.

It's particularly important that young people drink enough liquid before, during, and after exercise, because they can get dehydrated faster than adults doing the same amount of activity. Make sure they have access to plenty of water, diluted fruit juice, or low-fat milk, and encourage them to keep drinking, because children aren't always very good at monitoring their own hydration levels. With the right fuel, they will hopefully enjoy sports and exercise more and grow to be active and healthy adults with good habits for life.

# BOOSTING BREAKFASTS

# BANANA AND DATE BREAKFAST SHAKE

**SERVES 3**

A shot of slow-releasing energy from dates and bananas is a smart way to support your energy levels for a big run or competition. And a smoothie is great if you don't want to feel over-full but still want to get in the maximum amount of carbs while hydrating at the same time. I add some ice to a Thermos flask and take this shake with me for an energy boost on the go.

2 ripe bananas
8 dates (5 if using Medjool dates), pitted
2 cups almond milk

**1.** Break the bananas into chunks and put them into a blender with the dates and almond milk.

**2.** Blend on high speed until smooth. For an extra cold shake, add a couple of ice cubes to the blender and blitz again.

**3.** Pour into three glasses to serve.

| PER SERVING | |
|---|---|
| CALORIES | 196 |
| FAT (g) | 2.0 |
| SATURATED FAT (g) | 0.2 |
| CARBS (g) | 40.0 |
| SUGAR (g) | 38.0 |
| FIBER (g) | 4.0 |
| PROTEIN (g) | 2.0 |
| SODIUM (g) | 0.21 |

**VARIATIONS**
Add 1 tablespoon of cacao nibs for a chocolate hit and an injection of heart-healthy antioxidants. Swap the almond milk for cow's milk or yogurt if you want to up your protein levels post-exercise.

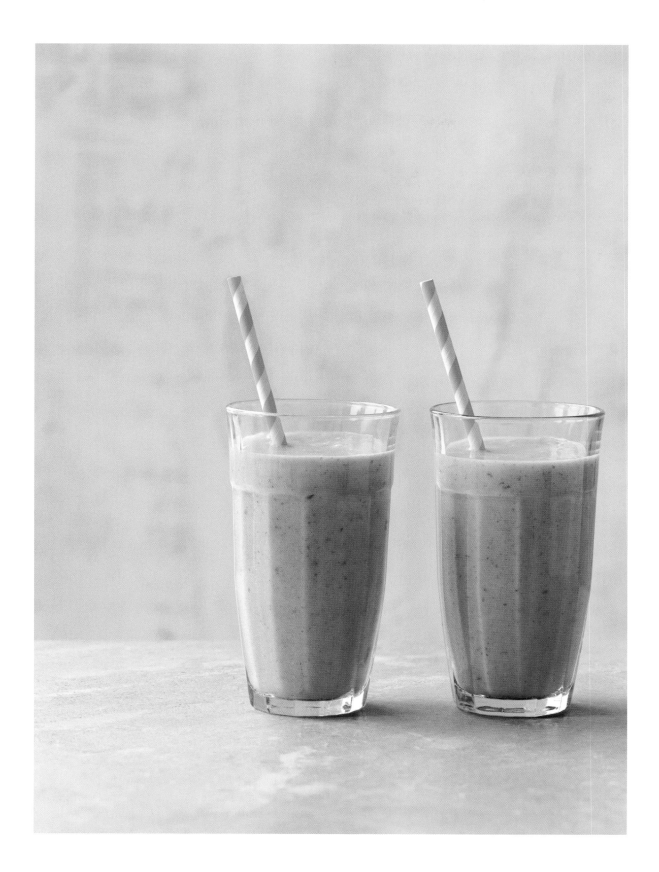

# FROZEN BERRY BREAKFAST BOWL

**SERVES 4**

The ladies in my life love a bowl of berries like this in the morning. I think it's because it tastes a lot like ice cream! Açai berries are one of the latest superfoods to reach our shores from South America and, among the many wondrous claims made of them, they are said to boost energy levels. So, no more excuses for staying in bed . . .

6 tablespoons açai juice, or ¼ cup açai powder
10½ ounces frozen berries, such as blueberries, raspberries, strawberries, or mixed berries
4 bananas, peeled, broken into pieces, and frozen for at least 2 hours
Water, coconut water, or apple juice, if needed
1 fresh banana
4 small handfuls of granola
2 handfuls of fresh blueberries

1. Put the açai juice or powder, frozen berries, and frozen bananas into a food processor or blender and process until smooth. If the mixture looks like it needs some help blending, add a small amount of liquid, a little at a time, to get it going. The mixture should blend to a soft-serve ice cream consistency rather than a smoothie consistency.

2. Transfer to serving bowls and top with sliced fresh banana, granola, and fresh blueberries. Serve immediately, before it starts to melt!

| PER SERVING | |
| --- | --- |
| CALORIES | 332 |
| FAT (g) | 12.0 |
| SATURATED FAT (g) | 4.0 |
| CARBS (g) | 43.0 |
| SUGAR (g) | 33.0 |
| FIBER (g) | 10.0 |
| PROTEIN (g) | 7.0 |
| SODIUM (g) | 0.04 |

**TO MAKE IT LEAN**
Leave out the açai juice or powder and replace it with an extra 3½ ounces of frozen berries if you're watching your weight.

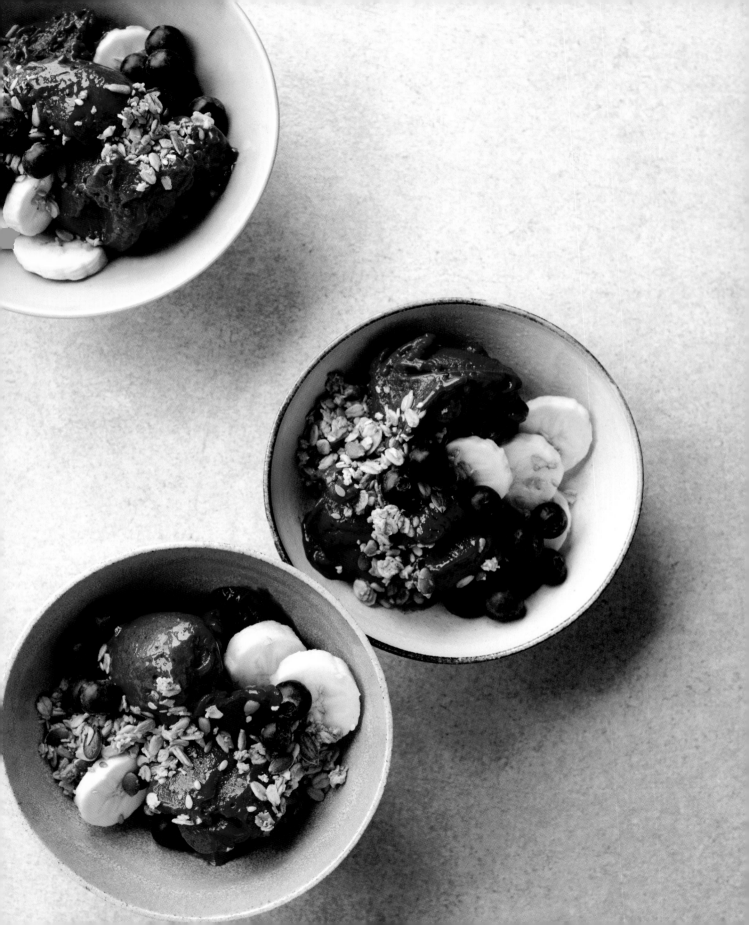

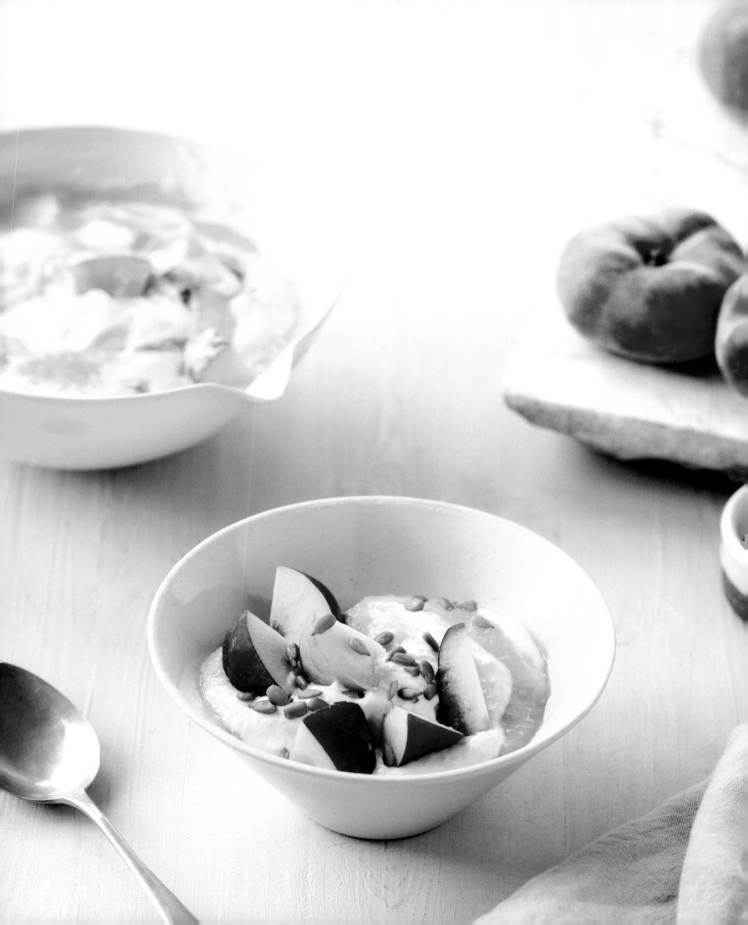

# YOGURT AND PEACH BOWL
**SERVES 4**

This is a really simple breakfast for the summer months, when peaches and nectarines are at their finest. The naturally occurring sugars in the fruit and honey are easily accessed and stored by the body for exertion in the day ahead, while the protein-rich yogurt helps stabilize energy levels so you don't have a sugar crash. You can use other fruits like plums or cherries, but avoid pineapple and kiwi, as they will make the yogurt curdle.

8 ripe peaches or nectarines, pitted
3 cups plain regular or Greek yogurt
2 tablespoons sunflower seeds

**1.** Peel 4 of the peaches and chop into chunks. Place the peaches into a blender and blitz until smooth, then set aside.

**2.** Swirl the peach purée through the yogurt to create a ripple effect. Cut the remaining peaches into bite-size pieces and stir half through the peach–yogurt mixture (do not blend). Divide the yogurt among four bowls.

**3.** Top each bowl with the remaining peach chunks and sprinkle the sunflower seeds over the top.

**FOR EXTRA ENERGY**
Sprinkle a handful of granola over the top of each bowl if you want to maximize your glycogen levels.

| PER SERVING | |
| --- | --- |
| CALORIES | 350 |
| FAT (g) | 23.0 |
| SATURATED FAT (g) | 13.0 |
| CARBS (g) | 20.0 |
| SUGAR (g) | 18.0 |
| FIBER (g) | 3.0 |
| PROTEIN (g) | 14.0 |
| SODIUM (g) | 0.31 |

# PEANUT BUTTER AND RASPBERRY JAM PANCAKES

**SERVES 6**

This is a simple gluten-free pancake recipe that provides lots of energy but won't slow you down. Make a big batch for the team and watch everyone devour them, knowing that they will be full of good things to draw on in the day ahead. It works just as well with other nut butters, so swap in cashew, hazelnut, or almond butter for a change.

1 cup peanut butter, smooth or crunchy
5 eggs
¼ cup plain yogurt
3 tablespoons Raspberry Chia Seed Jam (page 32), plus extra to serve
1 tablespoon canola oil
4 bananas, peeled and sliced
Maple syrup, to serve (optional)

**1.** Whisk the peanut butter, eggs, yogurt, and raspberry jam together in a bowl until well combined. The mixture should be a thick dropping consistency.

**2.** Place a large skillet over medium heat. Add a little of the oil and heat, swirling around the pan to coat. Add about 2 tablespoons of the mixture to the pan and spread it out thickly using the back of a spoon. Cook for 2 to 3 minutes, until lightly colored, then turn over and repeat on the other side.

**3.** Keep the pancakes warm in a low oven or wrapped in a kitchen towel while you cook the rest, adding more oil to the pan with each batch.

**4.** Serve with the sliced banana and extra dollops of jam, as well as a drizzle of maple syrup, if desired.

| PER SERVING | |
| --- | --- |
| CALORIES | 418 |
| FAT (g) | 29.0 |
| SATURATED FAT (g) | 7.0 |
| CARBS (g) | 18.0 |
| SUGAR (g) | 14.0 |
| FIBER (g) | 4.0 |
| PROTEIN (g) | 19.0 |
| SODIUM (g) | 0.60 |

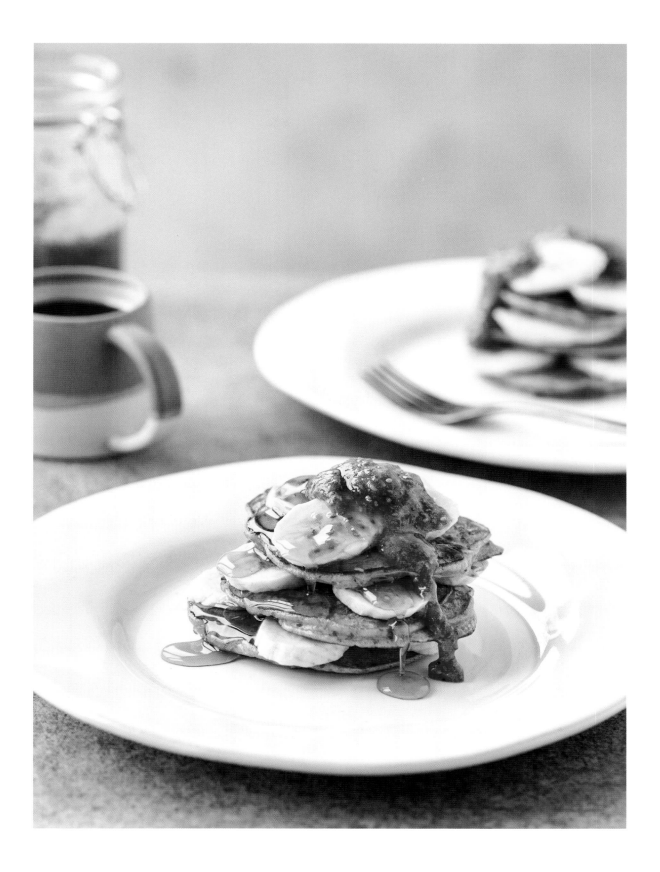

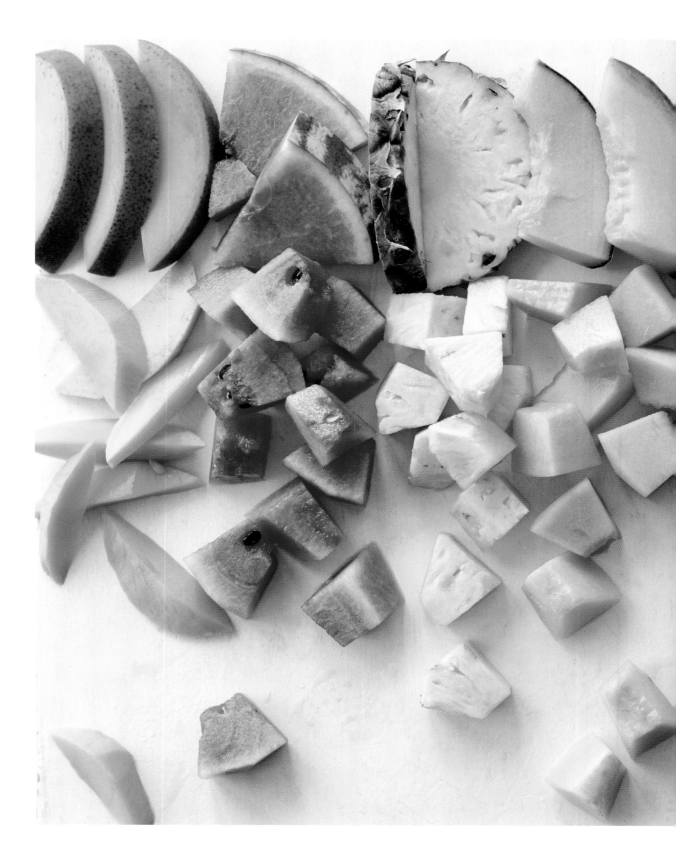

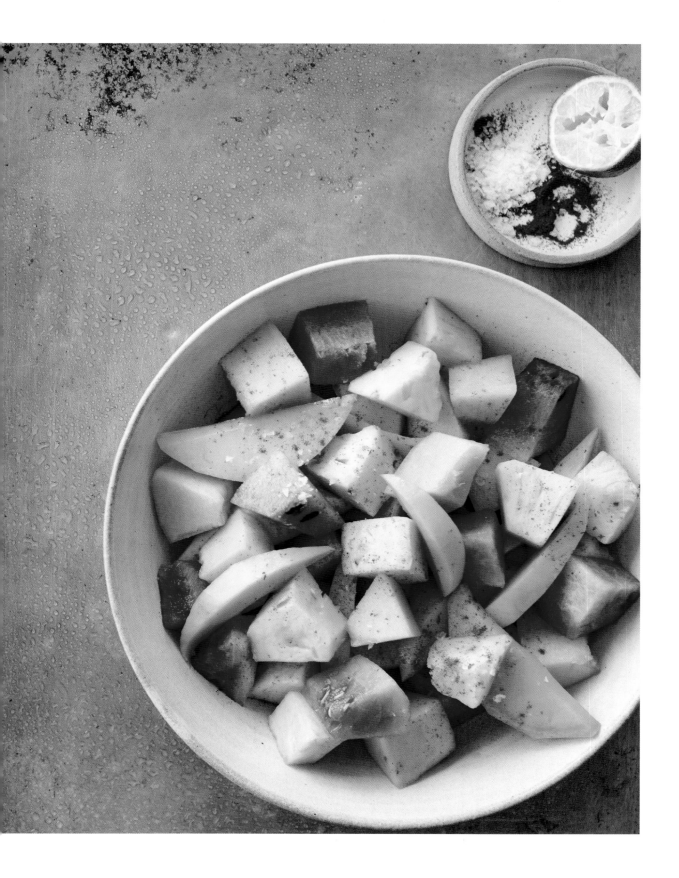

# MEXICAN FRUIT SALAD

**SERVES 8**

In LA, almost every street corner has a pushcart vendor selling some kind of food. One of the most popular things they sell is this refreshing fruit salad. It may sound strange to add salt and chile to fruit, but it's really tasty and oddly addictive. Plus, a pinch of chile powder in the morning is a great way to kick-start the day, and I love it before or after a morning run.

1 small ripe watermelon
1 ripe canteloupe
1 ripe mango
1 ripe pineapple
Juice of 1 lime
Fine sea salt
½ to 1 teaspoon chile powder (optional)

1. Prepare all the fruit, removing the skin and pits, and cut the flesh of each into similar bite-size pieces. Place in a large mixing bowl.

2. Squeeze the lime juice over the fruit pieces and mix well. Add a couple of pinches of salt and mix again so that everything is coated in a little citrus and salt.

3. Transfer to serving bowls, sprinkle each bowl with a little chile powder, if using, and serve immediately.

| PER SERVING | |
| --- | --- |
| CALORIES | 276 |
| FAT (g) | 1.0 |
| SATURATED FAT (g) | 0.1 |
| CARBS (g) | 58.0 |
| SUGAR (g) | 53.0 |
| FIBER (g) | 6.0 |
| PROTEIN (g) | 5.0 |
| SODIUM (g) | 0.12 |

**GOOD TO KNOW**
Watermelon is called watermelon for a reason—it's 92 percent water! Starting the day with fruit is such a good way to make sure your hydration levels are topped off before you get going.

# BAKED ENGLISH BREAKFAST

**SERVES 2**

A full English breakfast is usually a bit too high in fat to be a good idea after a workout, because fat can slow down the uptake of the vital protein you need for muscle repair after exertion. This baked version, however, is high in protein and lower in fat than a classic fry-up. It's also really easy to put together quickly, which is perfect for when you're in a hurry to refill the empty tank. A bacon medallion is the "eye" of a strip of back bacon, so it's the meaty part with the rind and fat removed. Back bacon is a product commonly found in the UK. As it can be difficult to find in US supermarkets, we've offered a lean bacon alternative here.

4 portobello mushrooms, brushed clean
3 medium tomatoes, halved
1 red onion, peeled and cut into 8 wedges
4 thyme sprigs, leaves only
2 tablespoons olive oil
Sea salt and freshly ground black pepper
6 smoked bacon medallions, or 6 strips of lean bacon, trimmed of fat
6 cups (7 ounces) baby spinach
4 eggs
2 thick slices of toast, to serve

**1.** Preheat the oven to 400°F.

**2.** Put the mushrooms, gill side up, and the tomatoes, cut side up, on a low-sided roasting pan. Scatter over the onion wedges and thyme leaves, then drizzle with the olive oil and sprinkle with salt and pepper.

**3.** Place the pan in the oven and roast for 20 minutes.

**4.** After 20 minutes, remove the pan from the oven and pour off any liquid that has been released by the mushrooms. Lay the bacon medallions or strips on top of the other ingredients, then return the pan to the oven to cook for 5 minutes.

**5.** Meanwhile, bring a kettle of water to a boil and put the spinach into a colander over your sink. When boiled, pour the water over the spinach to wilt it. When wilted, run it under cold water, then pick up the leaves in your hands and squeeze out as much excess liquid as you can.

**6.** Remove the pan from the oven and arrange the spinach leaves on top and around the other ingredients. Make four wells between the spinach and other ingredients and crack the eggs into them.

**7.** Put the pan back into the oven for another 8 minutes, then remove and serve the baked breakfast with thick slices of toast.

| PER SERVING | |
|---|---|
| CALORIES | 459 |
| FAT (g) | 25.0 |
| SATURATED FAT (g) | 5.0 |
| CARBS (g) | 14.0 |
| SUGAR (g) | 12.0 |
| FIBER (g) | 9.0 |
| PROTEIN (g) | 41.0 |
| SODIUM (g) | 0.57 |

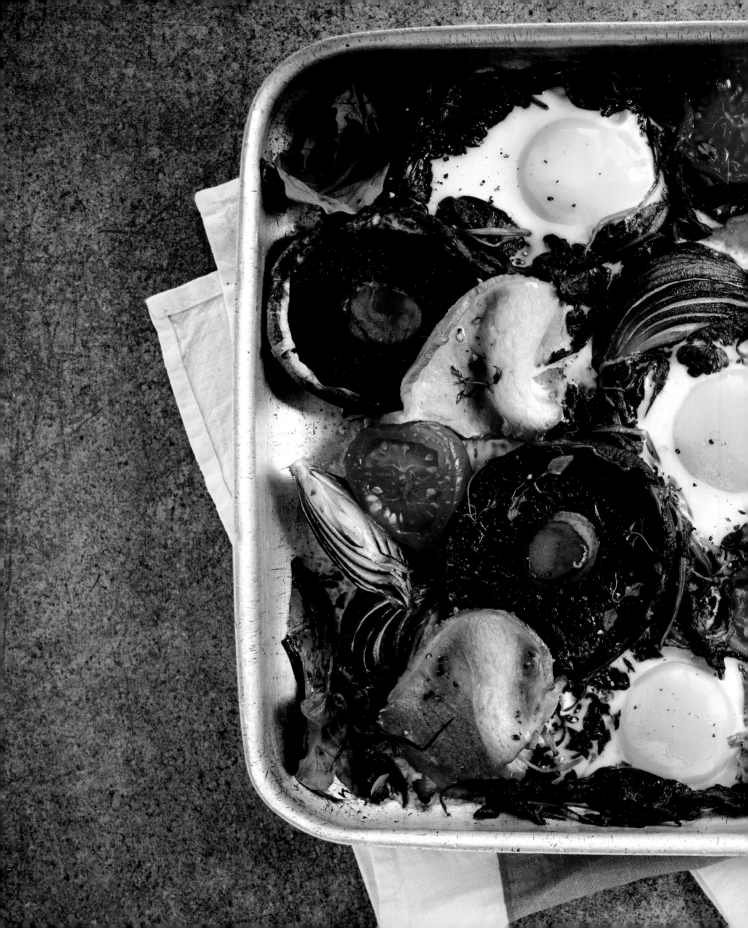

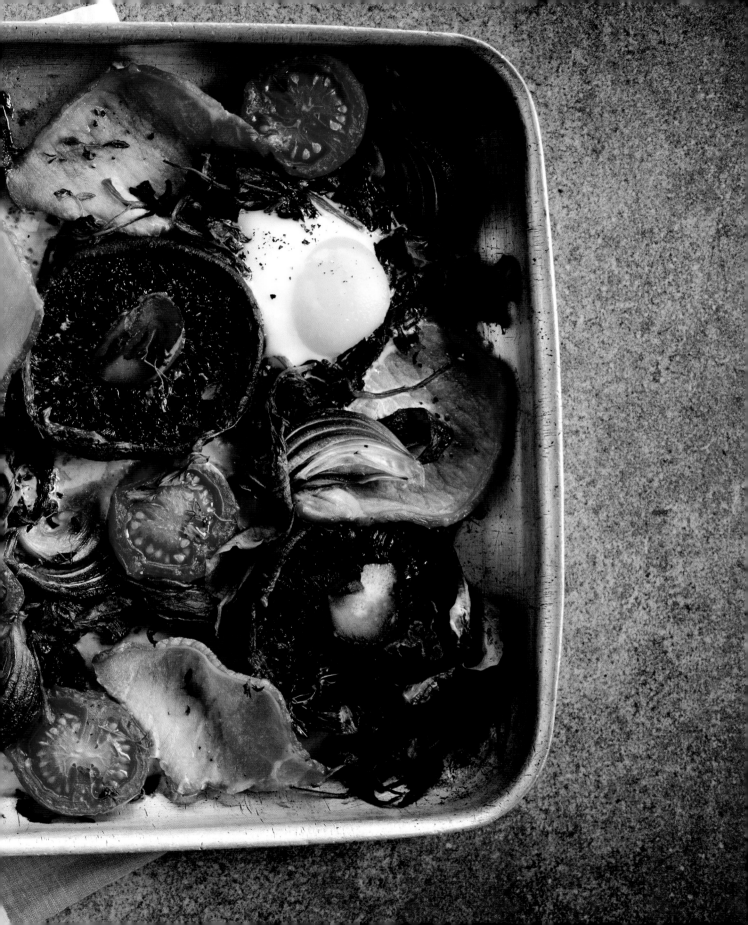

# BREAKFAST BURRITOS

**SERVES 4**

A wrap is the ideal portable breakfast if you have an early start. Make these burritos the night before and wrap them in foil to take with you, or enjoy them for brunch after a morning workout. They're packed with strong flavors, lean protein, and slow-releasing carbs to meet all your body's nutritional needs pre- or post-exertion.

**FOR THE SALSA**
1 large tomato, diced
½ small red onion, finely diced (use the remaining half below)
Juice of ½ lime
½ small bunch of cilantro, leaves and stems finely chopped
Dried chile flakes, to taste
Sea salt and freshly ground black pepper

**FOR THE BURRITOS**
Olive oil
½ small red onion (see above), diced
Sea salt
1 teaspoon ground cumin
1 (15-ounce) can black beans, adzuki beans, or pinto beans, drained
6 eggs
1 teaspoon chipotle paste (optional)
Freshly ground black pepper
4 large seeded wraps
1 ripe avocado, peeled, pitted, and sliced
Mexican hot sauce, such as Cholula (optional), to serve

**1.** Start by making the salsa. Mix all the ingredients together and season with salt and pepper. Taste and add more chile flakes or salt if needed. Set aside.

**2.** Place a large skillet over medium heat. Add a glug of oil and, once hot, add the diced onion with a pinch of salt. Sweat until translucent and softened, then add the cumin and continue to cook for 1 to 2 minutes, until fragrant.

**3.** Add the beans and stir until heated through.

**4.** Put the eggs into a bowl with the chipotle paste, if using, and beat together with a fork or whisk until well mixed. Season with a little black pepper. In a second pan over medium-low heat, scramble the eggs, stirring now and again until just beginning to set, then remove the pan from the heat and stir them into the beans.

**5.** Meanwhile, lay the wraps on four plates. Spoon the bean mixture in a horizontal line across the middle of each of the wraps and add a spoonful of salsa. Top with slices of avocado.

**6.** Fold the sides of each wrap inward, then roll from the bottom to the top until you have a log, wrapping the filling tightly inside.

**7.** Serve with a little hot sauce on the side, if desired.

| PER SERVING | |
| --- | --- |
| CALORIES | 432 |
| FAT (g) | 20.0 |
| SATURATED FAT (g) | 5.0 |
| CARBS (g) | 38.0 |
| SUGAR (g) | 4.0 |
| FIBER (g) | 9.0 |
| PROTEIN (g) | 21.0 |
| SODIUM (g) | 1.30 |

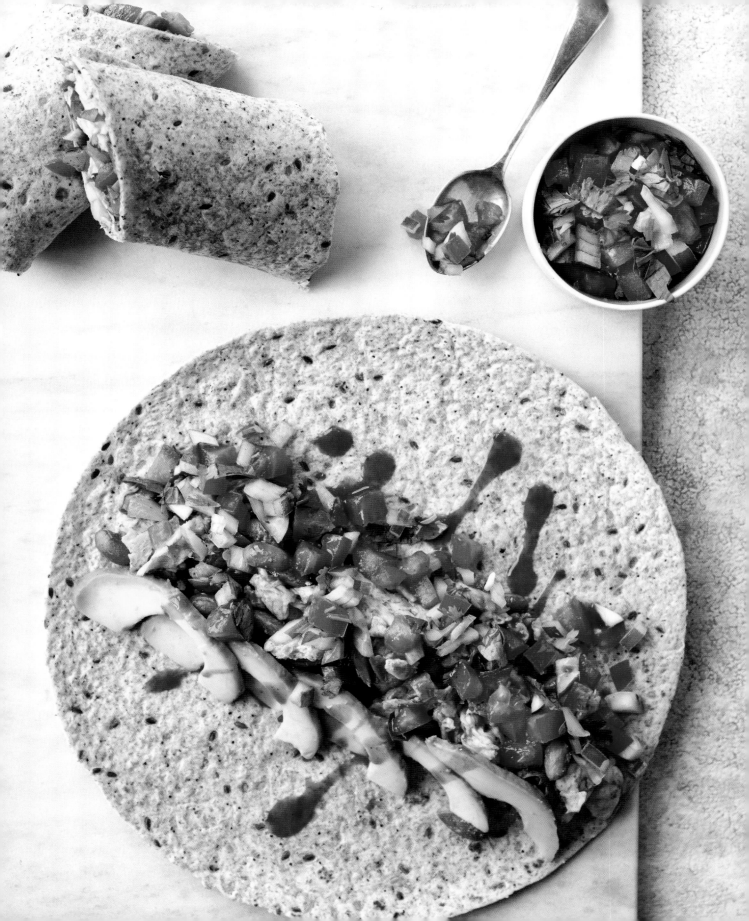

# HUEVOS RANCHEROS

**SERVES 2**

Huevos rancheros is a Mexican breakfast that makes a really substantial brunch before or after a big run or workout. It is easy to make and excellent for sharing with friends or family. If you don't like too much spice in the morning, leave the chipotle and red chiles out. Personally, I like the kick they give me.

2 (14-ounce) cans chopped tomatoes
1½ tablespoons olive oil
1 red onion, peeled and diced
1 garlic clove, peeled and sliced
1 green pepper, seeded and finely diced
1 dried chipotle chile
1 red chile, seeded and thinly sliced
Sea salt and freshly ground black pepper
4 eggs
2 tortillas, to serve
½ small bunch of cilantro, roughly chopped

1. Open one of the cans of tomatoes and tip the contents into a sieve to drain off approximately half the liquid. Set aside and use the juice for another dish (or in a bloody Mary!).

2. Place a medium skillet over medium-high heat and add the oil. When hot, add the red onion, garlic, green pepper, and the chipotle and red chiles. Cook the vegetables together for 3 minutes, or until just starting to soften.

3. Pour in the drained tomatoes as well as the complete can of tomatoes, season with salt and pepper, and bring to a boil. Reduce the heat to a simmer and cook for 2 minutes.

4. Make 4 wells in the tomato sauce and crack an egg into each one. Cover with a lid and cook for 8 minutes, or until the whites have set but the yolks are still runny.

5. Heat the tortillas according to the package instructions.

6. Serve the eggs and tomato sauce on top of the warm tortillas with a generous sprinkling of chopped cilantro.

| PER SERVING | |
| --- | --- |
| CALORIES | 379 |
| FAT (g) | 21.0 |
| SATURATED FAT (g) | 4.0 |
| CARBS (g) | 23.0 |
| SUGAR (g) | 21.0 |
| FIBER (g) | 7.0 |
| PROTEIN (g) | 21.0 |
| SODIUM (g) | 0.52 |

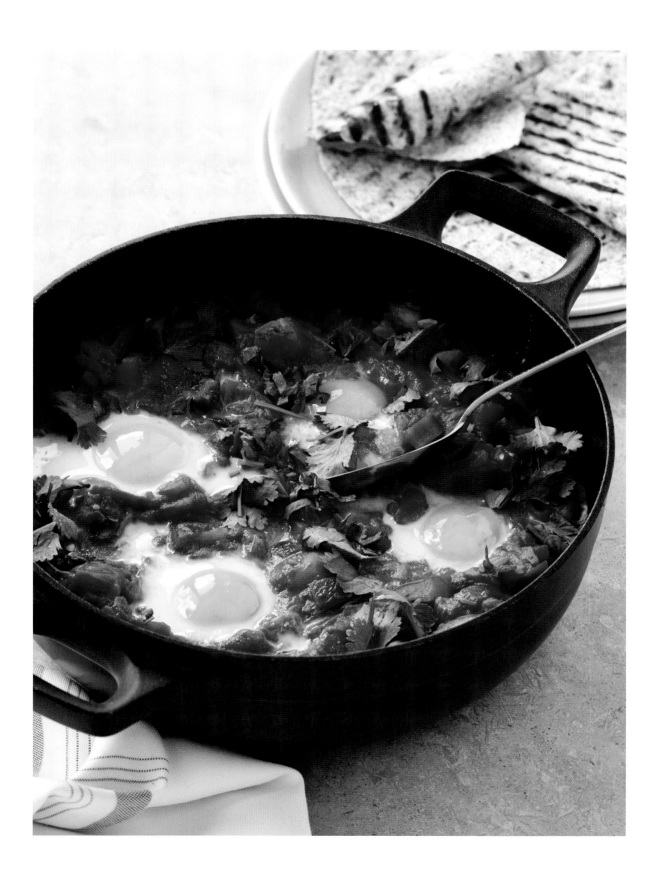

# LUNCHES FOR ACTIVE DAYS

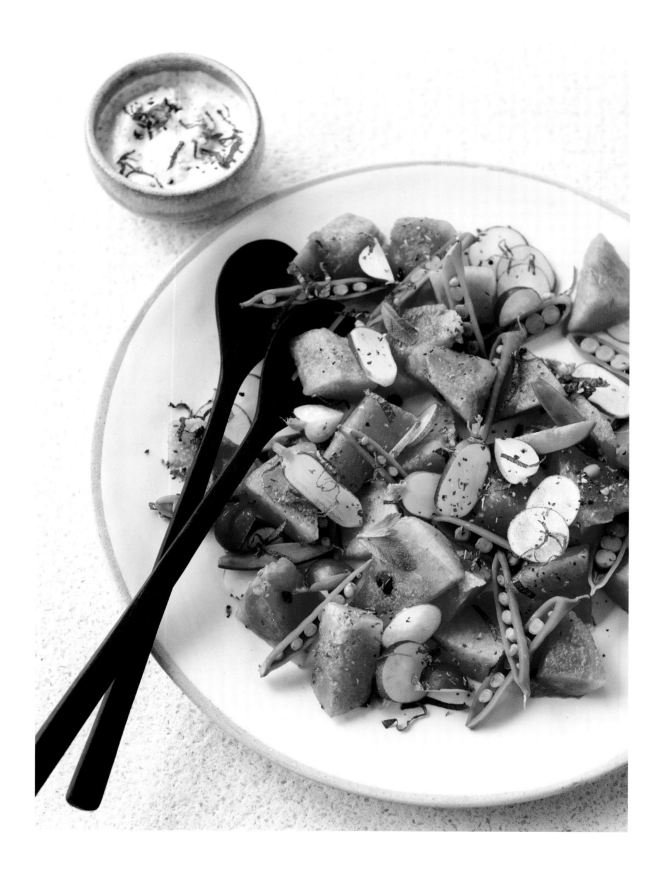

# WATERMELON, FETA, AND MINT SALAD
**SERVES 4**

Just because this salad sounds light and healthy doesn't mean it isn't packed with vital energy for active days. The naturally occurring sugars in the fruit, veg, and yogurt are easily accessed by the body but don't overload the system like more difficult-to-digest carbs. Don't make this too far in advance, as the salty cheese will draw the moisture out of the melon and it will lose its crispness.

## FOR THE DRESSING
2½ ounces feta cheese, drained and crumbled
½ cup plain yogurt
Dash of water or milk
1 tablespoon thinly sliced mint leaves
Freshly ground black pepper

## FOR THE SALAD
½ small watermelon, flesh cut into chunks
1 bunch of radishes, trimmed and sliced
3½ ounces sugar snap peas, trimmed and sliced
½ teaspoon dried oregano
½ small bunch of mint, leaves thinly sliced

**1.** To make the dressing, put the feta into a bowl and blend with a stick blender until smooth. Alternatively, put the feta into a bowl and mash with a fork.

**2.** Add the yogurt and mix well, add a dash of water or milk if needed, then stir in the mint leaves. Taste and season with a little pepper.

**3.** Arrange the watermelon, radishes, and sugar snap peas on a serving platter. Sprinkle over the dried oregano and the sliced mint leaves, then drizzle over the feta dressing before serving.

## FOR EXTRA PROTEIN
If you want to add some extra protein to this dish, a grilled tuna steak or some squid would be delicious, as would some shrimp, grilled chicken, or lamb kebabs.

| PER SERVING | |
|---|---|
| CALORIES | 275 |
| FAT (g) | 6.0 |
| SATURATED FAT (g) | 3.0 |
| CARBS (g) | 45.0 |
| SUGAR (g) | 39.0 |
| FIBER (g) | 3.0 |
| PROTEIN (g) | 9.0 |
| SODIUM (g) | 0.56 |

# VEGETABLE CARPACCIO, CANDIED PECAN, AND BLUE CHEESE SALAD

**SERVES 4**

This crunchy salad is stunning to look at as well as to eat, especially if you manage to get ahold of different colored heirloom beets. Choose a firmer blue cheese that crumbles easily, like Stilton, Roquefort, or Shropshire Blue, rather than a creamy dolcelatte or Auvergne. Serve with whole-wheat or pumpernickel bread for added carbohydrates.

**FOR THE CANDIED PECANS**
¾ cup pecan halves
1 tablespoon maple syrup
Pinch of salt

**FOR THE VEGETABLES**
3 raw beets, ideally different colors, such as yellow, purple, and candy striped, cleaned and peeled
1 green apple
Juice of 1 lemon
1 small bunch of radishes
1 head chicory
2 carrots
3 celery stalks, any leaves reserved
2½ ounces blue cheese, crumbled
Sea salt and freshly ground black pepper

**FOR THE WALNUT DRESSING**
2 tablespoons walnut oil
2 tablespoons extra virgin olive oil
Juice of 1 lemon
½ small bunch of chives, very finely chopped
Sea salt and freshly ground black pepper

| PER SERVING | |
|---|---|
| CALORIES | 377 |
| FAT (g) | 31.0 |
| SATURATED FAT (g) | 6.0 |
| CARBS (g) | 15.0 |
| SUGAR (g) | 13.0 |
| FIBER (g) | 6.0 |
| PROTEIN (g) | 8.0 |
| SODIUM (g) | 0.71 |

**1.** Preheat the oven to 350°F.

**2.** First, make the candied pecans: Toss the pecans in the maple syrup and season with a pinch of salt. Spread them in a single layer on a baking sheet and roast in the oven for 5 to 7 minutes, turning halfway through, until lightly toasted and caramelized. Watch the nuts carefully so they don't burn. Remove and leave to cool.

**3.** Meanwhile, prepare the vegetables. The best instrument for this recipe is a mandoline, but use a very sharp knife if you don't have one. Slice the beets into wafer-thin rounds and place in a large mixing bowl of cold water (if you are using purple beets, put them into a separate bowl to avoid staining).

**4.** Core the apple, then slice it into wafer-thin rounds and put them into the mixing bowl, adding the lemon juice to prevent them from turning brown.

**5.** Slice the radishes and chicory and add to the bowl.

**6.** Using a vegetable peeler, peel the carrots into long thin ribbons and put them into the bowl with the other vegetables.

**7.** Slice the celery very thinly on the diagonal.

**8.** Next, make the dressing: Whisk together the ingredients with a good pinch of salt and pepper.

**9.** When ready to serve, drain the vegetables and pat them dry with a clean dish towel or paper towels. Put them all into a dry mixing bowl, pour in the dressing, and toss gently to coat. Taste and add more seasoning as necessary.

**10.** Add the crumbled blue cheese and candied pecans and toss again to mix. Transfer to a serving dish and garnish with any reserved celery leaves before serving.

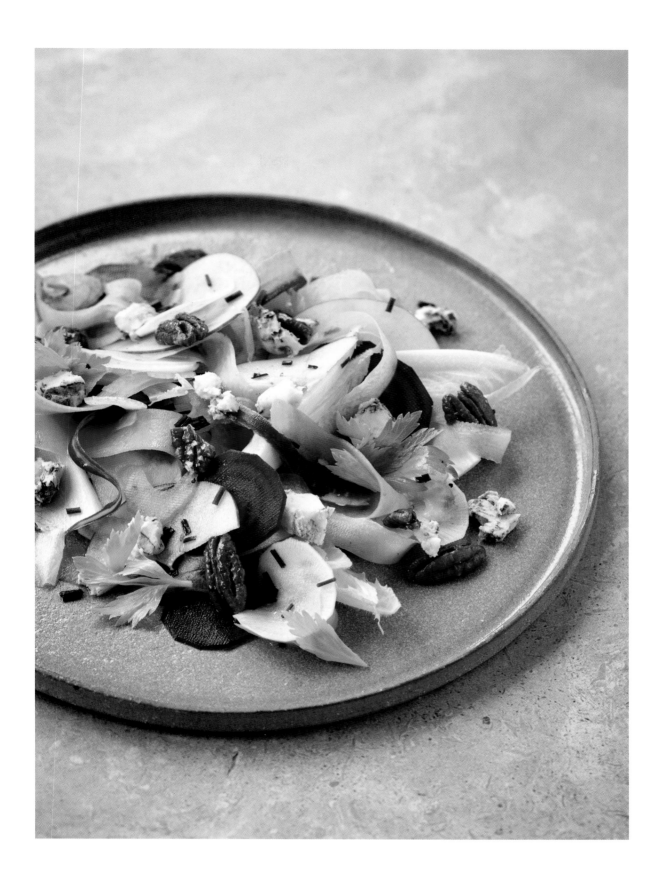

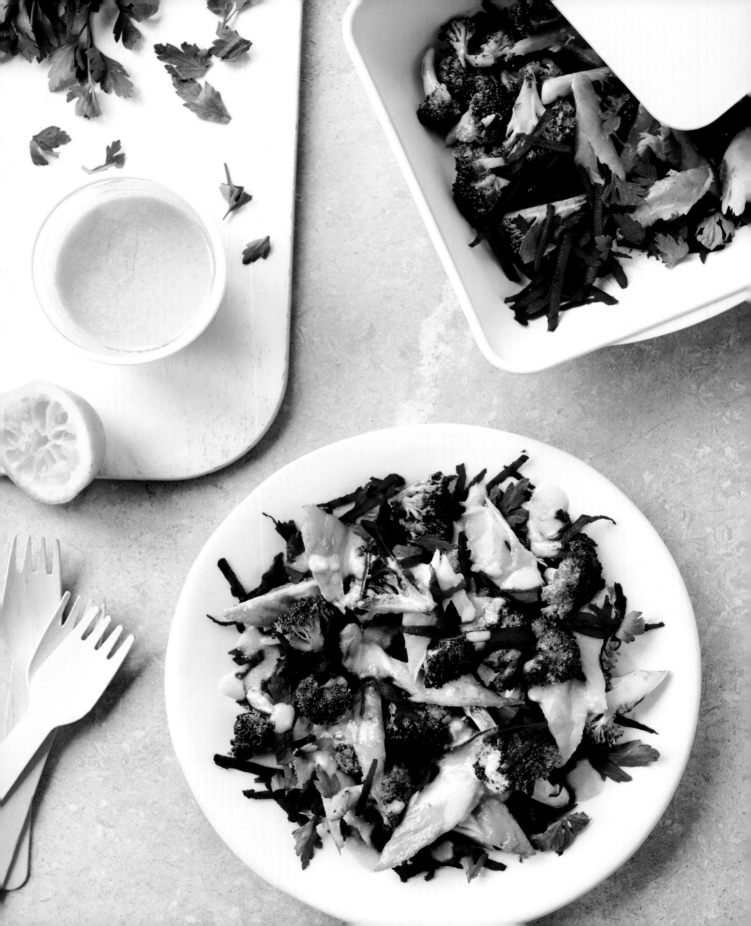

# SMOKED MACKEREL, BEET, AND BROCCOLI SALAD

**SERVES 4**

Beets are the gym-goer's secret weapon—studies show that eating beets and drinking their juice helps you stay the course that little bit longer. Serving them raw is surprisingly delicious, and it guarantees that none of the nutrients have been lost through cooking. You could keep the broccoli florets raw, too, but charring them does add a delicious caramelized flavor to the salad. This is a good protein-packed lunch to take with you for post-exercise replenishment.

1 medium head broccoli, cut into florets
Olive oil
Sea salt and freshly ground black pepper
14 ounces beets, peeled and grated
4 smoked mackerel fillets
¼ small bunch of parsley, leaves roughly chopped

**FOR THE DRESSING**
1 tablespoon prepared horseradish
Juice of ½ lemon
2 tablespoons extra virgin olive oil

**1.** Heat a large skillet over medium heat and add the broccoli florets. Drizzle with a little olive oil and season with salt and pepper. Toss to evenly coat the broccoli with oil. Leave the broccoli in the pan without stirring for 3 to 4 minutes, until lightly browned on one side. Turn and repeat on the other side. Once charred but still crunchy, remove from the heat.

**2.** Meanwhile, whisk together the ingredients for the dressing in a small bowl until combined. Taste and adjust the seasoning as necessary, adding more lemon juice if needed.

**3.** Put the grated beet onto a serving platter, scatter over the broccoli, and gently mix together. Flake over the smoked mackerel fillets, keeping an eye out for bones, then sprinkle with the chopped parsley and gently toss.

**4.** Drizzle with the dressing and serve immediately, or store covered in the fridge for up to 3 days.

**FOR EXTRA ENERGY**
Add a handful of cooked lentils, couscous, or another grain per person if you're carb-loading.

| PER SERVING | |
| --- | --- |
| CALORIES | 611 |
| FAT (g) | 44.0 |
| SATURATED FAT (g) | 8.0 |
| CARBS (g) | 12.0 |
| SUGAR (g) | 10.0 |
| FIBER (g) | 8.0 |
| PROTEIN (g) | 39.0 |
| SODIUM (g) | 3.08 |

# SUSHI SALAD BOWL

**SERVES 4**

This is a great way to get all the flavors of sushi without any of the hassle of making it. The seaweed isn't essential, but given that it provides an impressive amount of valuable nutrients as well as a mouth-pleasing umami hit, it is definitely worth experimenting with. Although this is very filling as it is, you can up the protein content by adding smoked or raw salmon, tuna, shrimp, or other flaked fish.

1 head broccoli, cut into small florets
2 tablespoons dried seaweed such as dulse fronds or wakame (if unavailable, replace with 3 crumbled sheets of nori)
2 cups cooked and cooled brown rice
1 cucumber, seeded and sliced
2 ripe avocados, peeled, pitted, and sliced
¼ cup pickled ginger, cut into strips
2 tablespoons sesame seeds, tan or white
½ small bunch of chives, finely chopped
2 tablespoons soy sauce
4 teaspoons brown rice vinegar
2 teaspoons toasted sesame oil

1. Blanch the broccoli florets by plunging them into a pot of boiling salted water for 2 minutes, or until the rawness has been removed but they are still crunchy. Refresh immediately in cold water to prevent further cooking. Chop into bite-size pieces.

2. Meanwhile, soak the dried seaweed in a bowl of warm water for 5 minutes, or until soft (if using crumbled nori, you do not need to soak it). Drain.

3. Divide the rice among four serving bowls, pushing it to one side so it takes up a quarter of the bowl. Add the cooled broccoli to another quarter. Add the cucumber and avocado in the same way, and then the seaweed. (If you're using crumbled nori, sprinkle it over the top with the sesame seeds in step 4.)

4. Sprinkle over the pickled ginger strips, sesame seeds, and chopped chives. Drizzle each bowl with some of the soy sauce and add the rice vinegar and sesame oil before serving.

| PER SERVING | |
| --- | --- |
| CALORIES | 411 |
| FAT (g) | 21.0 |
| SATURATED FAT (g) | 4.0 |
| CARBS (g) | 36.0 |
| SUGAR (g) | 5.0 |
| FIBER (g) | 12.0 |
| PROTEIN (g) | 14.0 |
| SODIUM (g) | 1.39 |

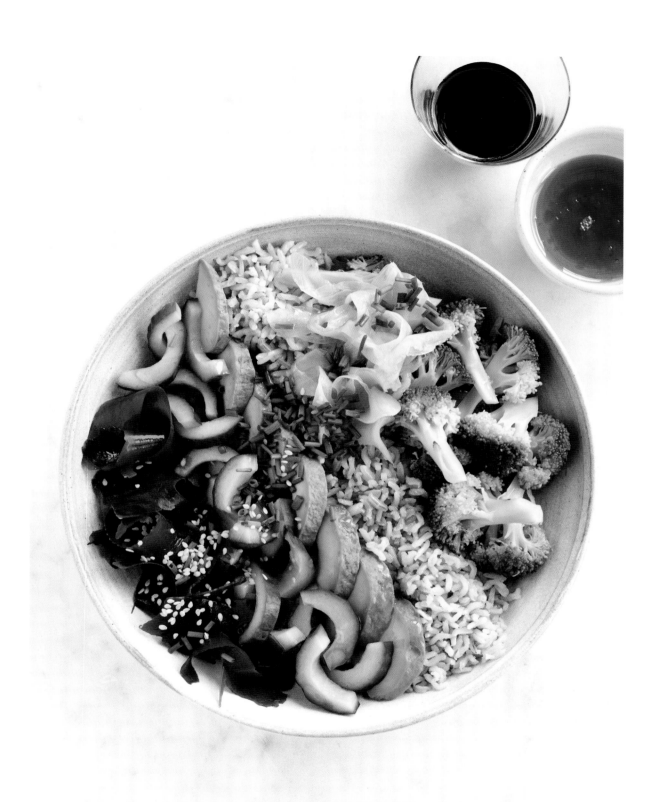

# VIETNAMESE CRISPY TOFU WRAP

**SERVES 4**

The flavors in this recipe are taken from the popular Vietnamese sandwich bánh mì, but I've ditched the meat in favor of baked, marinated tofu and replaced the white baguette with a whole-wheat wrap. Same great taste but better energy sources for exercise. The pickled vegetables and the sriracha yogurt dressing are both great things to have on standby in your fridge to perk up almost any meal.

**FOR THE PICKLED VEGETABLES**
½ cup rice wine vinegar
2 teaspoons agave syrup
1 carrot, peeled and julienned
½ daikon radish, julienned (if unavailable, use 6 radishes, trimmed and sliced)

**FOR THE VIETNAMESE TOFU**
1 (12-ounce) package firm tofu, drained
1 tablespoon fish sauce
Juice of ½ lime
2 teaspoons agave syrup
¼ cup plain yogurt
1 teaspoon sriracha sauce
4 large whole-wheat wraps
1 Little Gem lettuce, shredded
½ cucumber, julienned
½ small bunch of cilantro, leaves roughly torn

| PER SERVING | |
| --- | --- |
| CALORIES | 322 |
| FAT (g) | 10.0 |
| SATURATED FAT (g) | 3.0 |
| CARBS (g) | 37.0 |
| SUGAR (g) | 11.0 |
| FIBER (g) | 7.0 |
| PROTEIN (g) | 17.0 |
| SODIUM (g) | 1.88 |

**VARIATIONS**
You can change the flavor of the tofu by altering the marinade: try a little miso paste mixed with a dash of soy sauce and rice vinegar or a mixture of soy sauce and hoisin sauce. And if you really don't like tofu, you can swap it out for marinated chicken pieces or shrimp.

1. For the pickled vegetables, mix together the rice wine vinegar and agave syrup in a wide, shallow bowl, then stir in the carrot and radishes and cover. Leave to pickle for a minimum of 30 minutes and up to 48 hours in the refrigerator.

2. Preheat the oven to 350°F.

3. Put the tofu on a plate between two layers of paper towels and place a heavy object such as a cast-iron pan on top. Press for 20 minutes to remove excess liquid.

4. Once the tofu has been pressed, slice it into bite-size pieces.

5. Mix together the fish sauce, lime juice, and agave syrup and toss the tofu pieces in the marinade until each piece is coated.

6. Place the tofu in a single layer on a nonstick baking sheet and bake for 20 to 25 minutes, turning occasionally, until crisp and golden on all sides but still soft in the middle.

7. Meanwhile, mix together the yogurt and sriracha sauce until combined.

8. Once the tofu is cooked, remove the sheet from the oven. Spread a little of the sriracha yogurt onto each tortilla wrap, then scatter over some Little Gem lettuce, cucumber matchsticks, and cilantro leaves. Top with the baked tofu and add some pickled vegetables and a little of the pickling liquid.

9. Add a dollop of extra sriracha yogurt, then fold the sides of the tortilla inward and roll from the bottom to the top until you have a log, wrapping the filling tightly inside. Slice in half on the diagonal to serve.

# CALIFORNIAN "FRIED" CHICKEN SANDWICH

**SERVES 4**

As a family with four teenage children, we are always looking for healthy ways of preparing not-so-healthy fast-food favorites like pizza, burgers, and fried chicken. This recipe is brilliant because it looks and tastes like a fried chicken sandwich, with the satisfying crunch from the chicken and the creaminess of the mayo, but is actually made with baked chicken and a yogurt dressing. The kids love it, we know they're eating well, and everyone's happy.

½ cup whole-wheat flour
1 cup buttermilk (or 2 eggs, beaten)
8 cups puffed rice
Sea salt and freshly ground black pepper
2 teaspoons garlic powder
2 teaspoons onion powder or granulated onion
4 teaspoons paprika
1 teaspoon dried sage
8 mini chicken breast fillets
4 whole-wheat buns
1 ripe avocado, peeled, pitted, and sliced
½ head iceberg lettuce, shredded
Mexican hot sauce, such as Cholula (optional), to serve

**FOR THE YOGURT DRESSING**
⅓ cup plain Greek yogurt
½ garlic clove, crushed
1 teaspoon cider vinegar
Sea salt and freshly ground black pepper

1. Preheat the oven to 350°F.

2. Put the flour, buttermilk, and puffed rice into three shallow bowls. Season the flour with salt and pepper. Add the garlic powder, onion powder, paprika, and dried sage to the buttermilk and mix well. Crush the puffed rice with your hands so that the pieces are broken down slightly but not powdered.

3. Dip a piece of chicken into the flour so it is completely covered. Remove and shake off any excess, then dip into the buttermilk. Allow any excess buttermilk to drip off, then put the chicken pieces into the puffed rice. Turn over to make sure they are completely coated, then place on a baking sheet. Repeat with the remaining chicken pieces.

4. Put the sheet into the oven and bake for 25 to 30 minutes, until the chicken is golden and cooked through, turning halfway through cooking.

5. Meanwhile, make the yogurt dressing: Mix together the yogurt, crushed garlic, and vinegar with a little salt and pepper. Taste and add more vinegar if needed.

6. Slice open the buns and divide the avocado slices among them. Top with the shredded iceberg lettuce.

7. Once the chicken is cooked, place on top of the lettuce and spoon over dollops of the yogurt dressing, as well as a drizzle of hot sauce, if desired. Close the buns and serve immediately.

| PER SERVING | |
| --- | --- |
| CALORIES | 510 |
| FAT (g) | 13.0 |
| SATURATED FAT (g) | 4.0 |
| CARBS (g) | 67.0 |
| SUGAR (g) | 10.0 |
| FIBER (g) | 8.0 |
| PROTEIN (g) | 27.0 |
| SODIUM (g) | 1.30 |

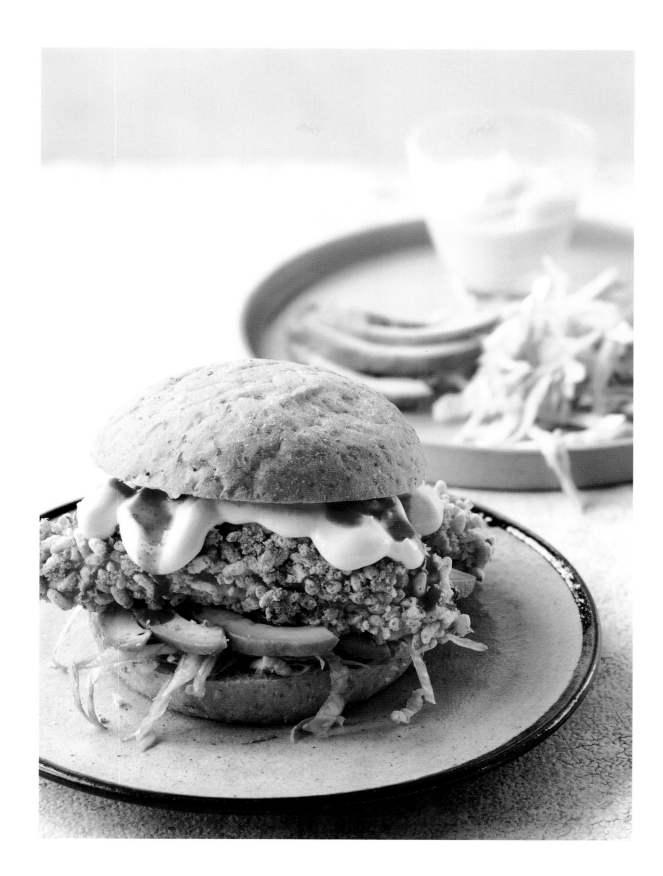

# CARB-LOADING FOR THE NIGHT BEFORE

# SAKE AND MISO STEAMED MUSSELS WITH SOBA NOODLES

**SERVES 4**

This is a Japanese take on the French classic moules marinières but without all the cream. Soba noodles are made from buckwheat flour, which is naturally fat- and gluten-free and provides lots of starchy carbohydrates for filling up the tank before a challenge. The noodles soak up all the delicious juices brilliantly, but miso is quite salty, so make sure you drink plenty of water at the same time. Also, the remains of the bottle of sake would be delicious served with this dish if you aren't running a marathon the following day!

4½ pounds fresh mussels
7 ounces soba noodles
4 ounces broccolini
1 tablespoon neutral oil, such as peanut
1 shallot, peeled and thinly sliced
¾-inch piece of fresh ginger, peeled and grated
2 garlic cloves, peeled and sliced
1 tablespoon miso paste
1 cup sake

1. To test that the mussels are okay to eat, place them in a sink or a large bowl of cold water. Throw away any that do not close when tapped against a hard surface. Drain the mussels and remove the beards.

2. Fill a medium saucepan with hot water and bring to a boil. Add the soba noodles and cook for 4 minutes, then add the broccolini. After 2 to 3 minutes, taste the soba noodles and, if done (tender but not soft or soggy), drain in a colander and divide among four serving bowls with the cooked broccolini.

3. Meanwhile, to cook the mussels, place a large heavy-bottomed casserole dish or saucepan with a tight-fitting lid over medium heat. Add the oil and, once hot, cook the shallot, ginger, and garlic for 2 minutes, or until the shallot begins to soften.

4. Add the miso paste and stir. Increase the heat, then add the sake and stir into the paste. Bubble for 2 minutes to burn off the alcohol, then tip in the mussels. Stir the mussels to coat them in the liquid, then put the lid on and cook for 3 to 4 minutes, shaking the pan occasionally, until all the mussels are open. Discard any that have not opened after cooking.

5. Divide the mussels and the cooking liquor among the four bowls of noodles and serve immediately.

| PER SERVING | |
| --- | --- |
| CALORIES | 439 |
| FAT (g) | 7.0 |
| SATURATED FAT (g) | 1.0 |
| CARBS (g) | 43.0 |
| SUGAR (g) | 1.0 |
| FIBER (g) | 1.0 |
| PROTEIN (g) | 34.0 |
| SODIUM (g) | 2.75 |

**GOOD TO KNOW**
Mussels are a valuable source of energizing iron—in fact, they contain more iron than red meat!

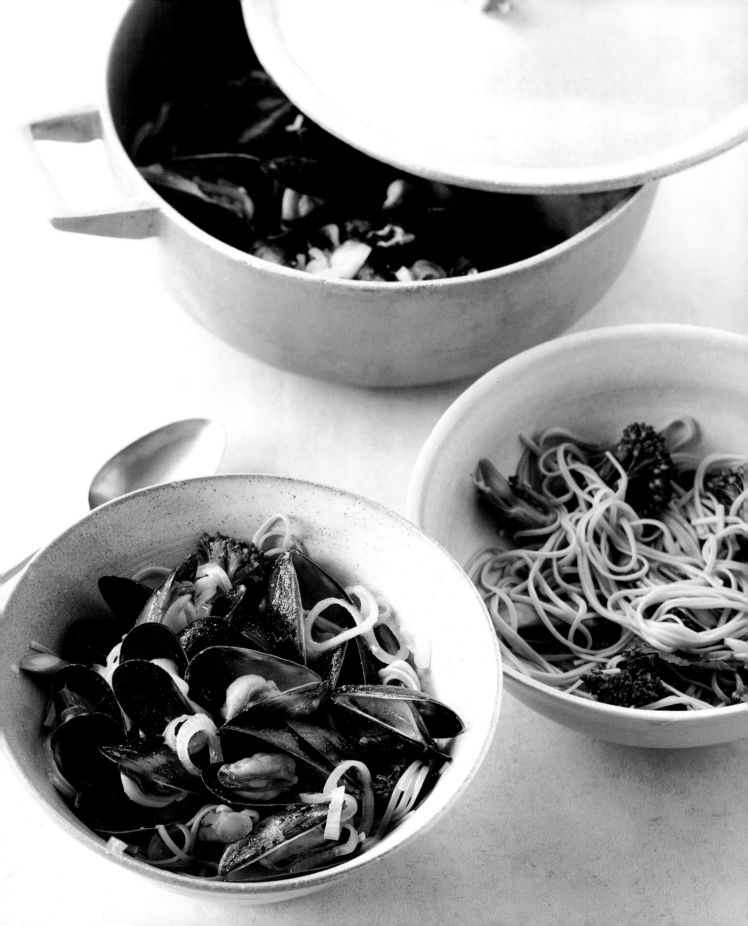

# SOUTHERN INDIAN FISH CURRY

**SERVES 6**

This is a lightly spiced, creamy curry with a delicate sweet-and-sour flavor that is popular in southern regions of India. Serve with boiled basmati or brown rice for a perfectly balanced pre-exercise meal. Coconut is rich in a certain type of saturated fat that is metabolized more rapidly than that from animal sources—this means coconut is a useful energy source for endurance sports.

½ tablespoon neutral oil, such as peanut
2 onions, peeled and thinly sliced
Sea salt
2 teaspoons mustard seeds
1 teaspoon ground turmeric
2 teaspoons ground cumin
1¼-inch piece of fresh ginger, peeled and grated
1 to 2 long red chiles, seeded and finely
   chopped, to taste
1 (13.5-ounce) can reduced-fat coconut milk
1 to 2 tablespoons tamarind paste or watered-down
   tamarind block (see tip on page 151)
Freshly ground black pepper
1 small eggplant, cut into bite-size pieces
2 carrots, chopped into bite-size rounds
7 ounces green beans, topped and tailed
   and cut in half
1½ pounds meaty white fish (such as cod, pollock,
   or haddock), cut into bite-size pieces

**TO SERVE**
Coconut and Ginger Brown Rice (see opposite)
2 tablespoons desiccated coconut, toasted (optional)

| PER SERVING | |
| --- | --- |
| CALORIES | 342 |
| FAT (g) | 8.0 |
| SATURATED FAT (g) | 5.0 |
| CARBS (g) | 42.0 |
| SUGAR (g) | 7.0 |
| FIBER (g) | 5.0 |
| PROTEIN (g) | 23.0 |
| SODIUM (g) | 0.22 |

**1.** Place a large, shallow saucepan or a high-sided skillet over medium heat and add the oil. Once hot, add the sliced onions with a pinch of salt and sauté for 8 to 10 minutes, until completely softened.

**2.** Add the spices and continue to cook for an additional minute, or until you can really smell them, then add the ginger and chiles and stir over the heat for an additional minute.

**3.** Add the coconut milk, tamarind paste, and 1¾ cups of water (use the empty coconut milk can to measure the 1¾ cups). Season with salt and pepper, stir well, and bring to a simmer.

**4.** Once the sauce is simmering, add the eggplant and continue to cook for 5 minutes, then add the carrots and simmer for 10 to 15 minutes, until the carrots and eggplant are tender and the sauce has thickened a little.

**5.** Add the green beans and cook for an additional 3 minutes, then add the fish. Stir well to coat, then cook for 3 to 4 minutes, until the fish is just cooked through. Taste and adjust the seasoning as necessary.

**6.** Serve the curry with the rice in warmed serving bowls, sprinkled with toasted desiccated coconut, if using.

# COCONUT AND GINGER BROWN RICE

**SERVES 6 AS A SIDE**

This rich and fragrant rice is delicious with curries or as a side to any Asian main course, and it makes a great change from plain boiled rice. Cooking the rice in coconut milk does increase the level of saturated and overall fat in the dish, but there are advantages to using coconut that make this an excellent choice for a pre-event supper.

1 tablespoon canola oil
1 small onion, peeled and finely diced
Sea salt
1¼-inch piece of fresh ginger,
    peeled and grated
1 teaspoon ground turmeric
1½ cups brown basmati rice
1 (13.5-ounce) can reduced-fat coconut milk
Chopped cilantro, to serve (optional)

1. Place a medium heavy-bottomed saucepan over medium heat. Add the canola oil and, once hot, add the finely diced onion with a pinch of salt. Cook for 5 to 6 minutes, until softened.

2. Add the ginger and turmeric and continue to cook for 2 minutes, stirring everything together. Then stir in the rice, making sure it is well coated in the flavored oil.

3. Pour in the coconut milk and 1¾ cups of boiling water and bring to a simmer. Simmer for 5 minutes, then reduce the heat to low and cover with a lid. Cook for an additional 30 to 35 minutes, until the rice is tender and the liquid has been absorbed.

4. Remove the rice from the heat, fluff with a fork, and season with a pinch of salt if needed. Serve immediately, sprinkled with cilantro, if using.

**HOW TO USE UP LEFTOVER RICE**
Leftover rice can be stir-fried the next day with added vegetables, eggs, meat, shrimp, or tofu for a delicious lunch or supper.

| PER SERVING | |
| --- | --- |
| CALORIES | 289 |
| FAT (g) | 9.0 |
| SATURATED FAT (g) | 5.0 |
| CARBS (g) | 45.0 |
| SUGAR (g) | 2.0 |
| FIBER (g) | 2.0 |
| PROTEIN (g) | 6.0 |
| SODIUM (g) | 0.0 |

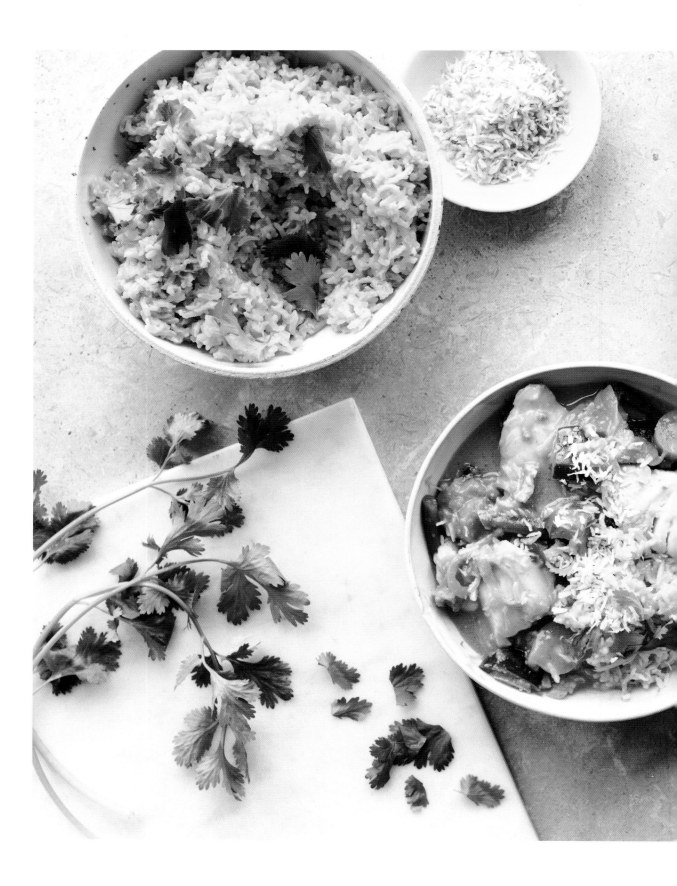

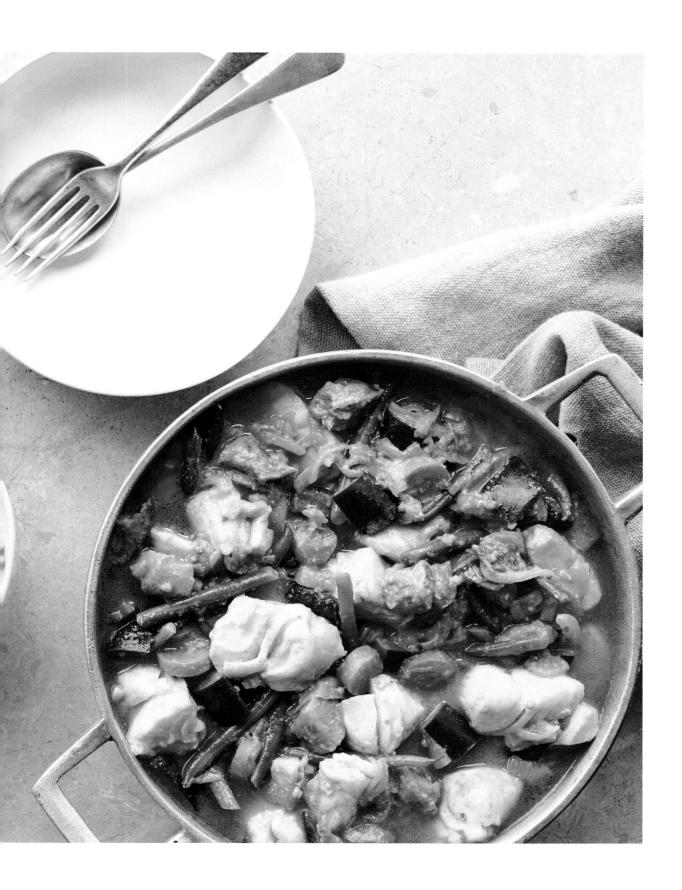

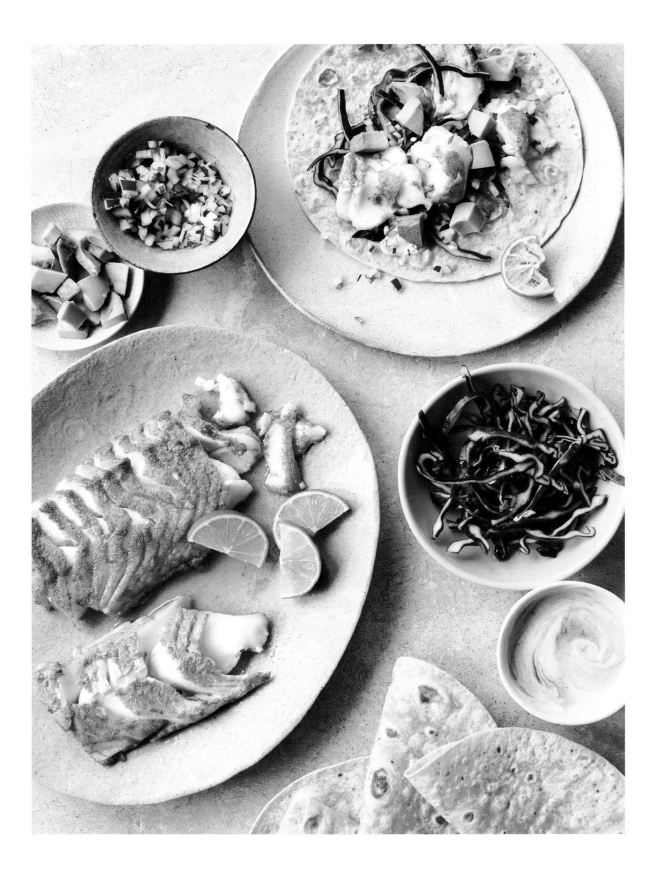

# SPICED FISH TACOS

**SERVES 4**

We love tacos in my house, particularly because everyone has their individual preferences when it comes to Mexican food. My son, Jack, for example, loves things really, really hot, while his twin sister, Holly, likes to keep it much milder. Therefore, we put all the different components on the table and get everyone to help themselves to their own perfect taco. These are brilliant to serve before a race or match day because each individual can eat as many tacos as they need depending on whether they are taking part or not.

½ cup plain yogurt
½ tablespoon chipotle paste, or to taste
¼ small red cabbage, finely shredded
1 small red onion, peeled and finely diced
1 ripe avocado, peeled, pitted, and roughly chopped
2 limes, cut into wedges
12 small soft corn tortillas or 4 large ones
2 teaspoons ground cumin
1 teaspoon smoked paprika
1½ tablespoons rice flour or all-purpose flour
Sea salt and freshly ground black pepper
10 ounces meaty white fish fillets, skin and pinbones removed
Coconut oil or neutral oil, such as peanut

1. Mix together the yogurt and chipotle paste. If you prefer a slightly hotter chipotle sauce, add a little more than half a tablespoon. Put into a small serving bowl and set aside.

2. Put the shredded cabbage, red onion, avocado, and lime wedges each in their own bowls and set aside.

3. Place a large skillet over medium heat. Have a bowl of water next to the pan and put the tortillas into the pan two at a time for 2 minutes to heat through. As they heat, sprinkle them with a little water by dipping your fingers into the bowl of water and flicking it at the tortillas. Turn the tortillas halfway through, then wrap them in a clean dish towel to stay warm while you heat the rest.

4. Mix together the ground cumin, smoked paprika, and flour and season with a pinch of salt and pepper. Dip the fish fillets into the spiced flour, making sure they are well covered.

5. Heat 1 tablespoon of coconut oil in the skillet and, once hot, fry the fish for 2 to 4 minutes on each side (depending on thickness of the fillets), until just cooked through. Remove from the heat.

6. Flake the fish into bite-size chunks and put them onto a serving plate. Bring to the table with the vegetables, sauce, limes, and tortillas and get everyone to build their own tacos.

**VARIATIONS**

This is a great recipe for trying out new varieties of fish that you might not usually buy. Try pollock or hake to make a change from the usual haddock or cod.

| PER SERVING | |
| --- | --- |
| CALORIES | 575 |
| FAT (g) | 19.0 |
| SATURATED FAT (g) | 5.0 |
| CARBS (g) | 73.0 |
| SUGAR (g) | 5.0 |
| FIBER (g) | 4.0 |
| PROTEIN (g) | 26.0 |
| SODIUM (g) | 2.86 |

# CHICKEN AND CHICKPEA TAGINE

**SERVES 4**

As well as carbohydrates, my training diet focuses on lean protein such as chicken and fish. It's a simple menu that can get quite repetitive, which is why I enjoy rich braises like this tagine. It's deeply tasty, very filling, and easy to digest. The chickpeas and couscous are a brilliant source of carbohydrates and the spices keep my taste buds from getting bored—it's a win-win.

5 cups chicken stock
1¾ cups couscous
Pinch of saffron
Olive oil
2¼ pounds chicken thighs, skin removed
2 onions, peeled and diced
2 garlic cloves, peeled and thinly sliced
1 cinnamon stick
2 teaspoons ground coriander
1 teaspoon ground turmeric
2 preserved lemons, finely chopped
2 (15-ounce) cans chickpeas, drained and rinsed
½ cup pitted black olives, halved
2 spring onions, trimmed and thinly sliced
6 radishes, trimmed and quartered
½ bunch of parsley, roughly chopped
Sea salt and freshly ground black pepper

1. Put the chicken stock into a saucepan and bring to a boil.

2. Tip the couscous into a large bowl and pour over 2 cups of the boiling chicken stock. Cover the bowl with plastic wrap and leave to stand. Add the saffron to the remaining chicken stock and leave to infuse.

3. Place a large casserole over medium–high heat and add a little olive oil. When hot, add half the chicken thighs and cook until golden brown all over, then remove them to a plate. Add a little more oil if needed, then repeat the process with the remaining chicken thighs.

4. Reduce the heat under the casserole to medium and add the onions, garlic, and cinnamon stick. Sauté for 8 to 10 minutes, until the onions are very soft and have turned translucent. If the onions are sticking to the bottom of the pan, add a splash of water rather than more oil to deglaze.

5. Stir in the coriander, turmeric, and chopped preserved lemon and continue to sauté for 1 minute, stirring occasionally.

6. Return the browned chicken thighs to the pan, then pour over the infused chicken stock. Bring to a boil, then reduce to a simmer and cook for 20 minutes.

7. After 20 minutes, add the chickpeas and olives to the casserole and continue to cook for an additional 15 minutes, or until the chicken is cooked through and the chickpeas are soft.

8. Meanwhile, remove the plastic wrap from the top of the couscous and add the sliced spring onions, radishes, a drizzle of olive oil, and half the chopped parsley. Season well with salt and pepper.

9. Stir the remaining chopped parsley into the tagine and serve with the couscous.

| PER SERVING | |
| --- | --- |
| CALORIES | 902 |
| FAT (g) | 27.0 |
| SATURATED FAT (g) | 5.0 |
| CARBS (g) | 101.0 |
| SUGAR (g) | 8.0 |
| FIBER (g) | 16.0 |
| PROTEIN (g) | 56.0 |
| SODIUM (g) | 1.09 |

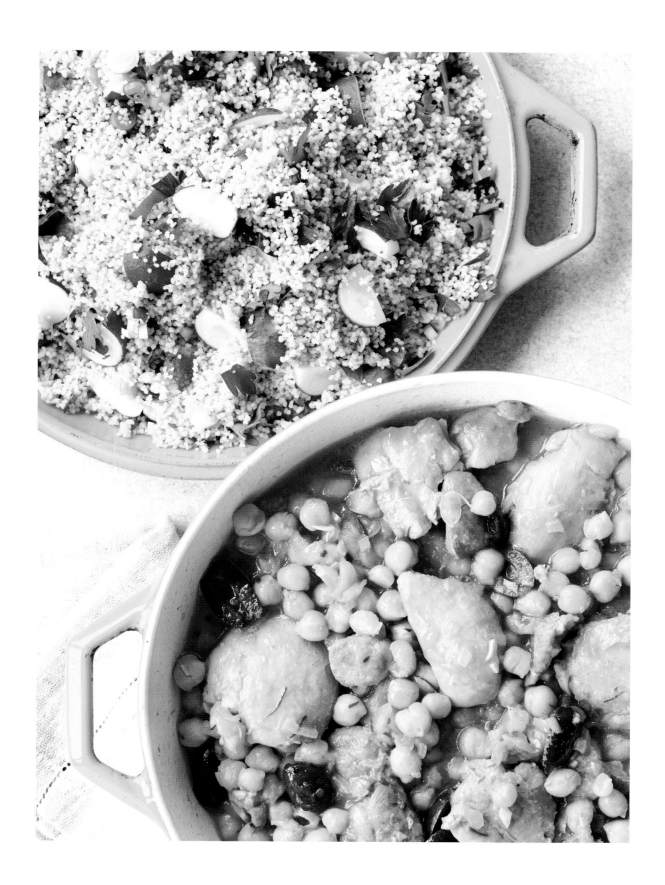

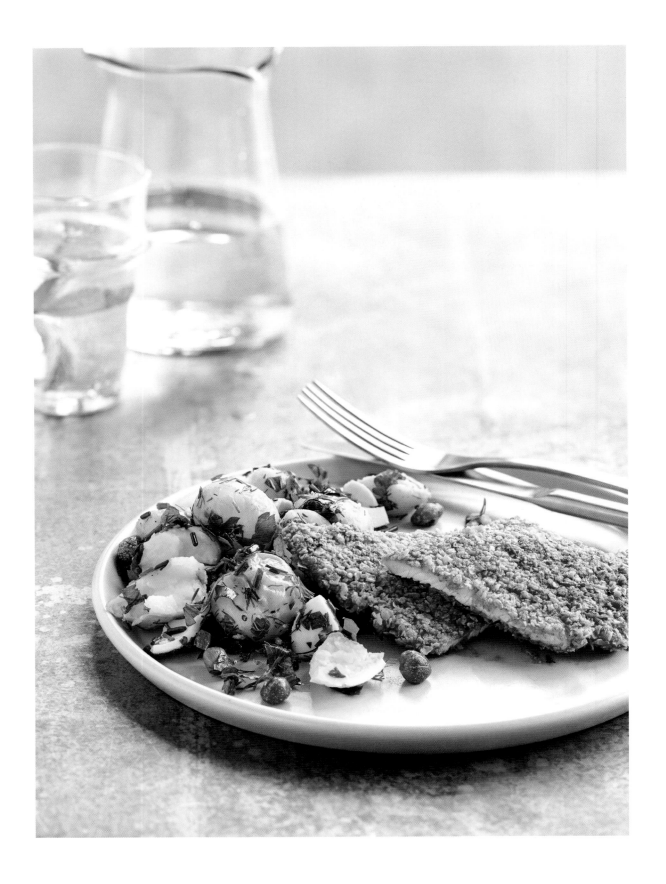

# CRISPY SPICED TURKEY
# WITH EGG AND POTATO SALAD

**SERVES 2**

Finding ways to load up on carbohydrates without relying on pasta and baked potatoes can be challenging. This crispy turkey is coated with oats and served with an herby new potato salad that will make carb-loading a doddle. When pounding the turkey, keeping its shape isn't as important as getting an even thickness all over, so don't worry if it looks a bit strange.

2 turkey breasts, skin removed
1½ cups rolled oats
1 tablespoon sweet smoked paprika
2 eggs
⅓ cup flour
Sea salt and freshly ground black pepper
10 ounces new potatoes
3 tablespoons olive oil
2 tablespoons roughly chopped dill
2 tablespoons roughly chopped parsley
2 tablespoons roughly chopped chives
2 teaspoons capers
Arugula leaves, to serve

**1.** Lay a piece of plastic wrap over your cutting board and place a turkey breast on top. Lay a second piece of plastic wrap over the top and, using a meat mallet or rolling pin, pound the breast until it is about ⅓ inch thick all over. Repeat this process with the second breast.

**2.** Mix the oats with the smoked paprika, then scatter them over a large plate.

**3.** Crack one of the eggs into a shallow bowl and beat with a fork. Pour the flour onto a second plate and season well with salt and pepper.

**4.** Dip the flattened breasts into the flour one at a time, then dip them into the egg and, finally, coat them in the spiced oats. Keep the breasts in the fridge while you prepare the potatoes.

**CONTINUED ON PAGE 240**

| PER SERVING | |
| --- | --- |
| CALORIES | 859 |
| FAT (g) | 32.0 |
| SATURATED FAT (g) | 6.0 |
| CARBS (g) | 80.0 |
| SUGAR (g) | 3.0 |
| FIBER (g) | 12.0 |
| PROTEIN (g) | 57.0 |
| SODIUM (g) | 0.62 |

CONTINUED FROM PAGE 239

5. Bring a pan of water to a boil, add the potatoes, and cook for 5 minutes, then add the second egg and continue to cook for 10 minutes, or until the potatoes are cooked through.

6. Drain the egg and potatoes in a colander, then immediately run the egg under cold running water to cool it down.

7. When the potatoes are well drained, tip them into a large bowl. When cool enough to handle, peel and finely chop the egg and add it to the potatoes. Give them a rough stir with a fork to break open some of the potatoes, then, while still warm, pour in 1 tablespoon of the olive oil, the chopped dill, parsley, chives, and capers along with a good pinch of salt and pepper. Toss everything gently together, then set aside.

8. Place a large, nonstick skillet over medium–high heat and add the remaining olive oil. When it is hot, carefully slide the coated turkey breasts into the pan and cook for 4 minutes on each side, or until you are sure they are cooked through.

9. Serve the turkey with the salad and a handful of arugula leaves.

# SWEET POTATO CHIPS WITH CHERMOULA

**SERVES 4 AS A SIDE**

As well as being carbohydrate-rich, sweet potatoes have many health benefits that white potatoes do not—for example, they have more fiber and vitamins A and C than the common spud. Leaving the skin on and baking these chips also makes them better for you than unhealthy French fries. Chermoula is a punchy North African sauce that goes really well with the sweetness of the sweet potatoes, but leave it out if it clashes with the rest of your menu. These are great with the Californian "Fried" Chicken Sandwich on page 224 or with steak, burgers, or sausages.

3 sweet potatoes, scrubbed
1 tablespoon olive oil
Sea salt and freshly ground black pepper

**FOR THE CHERMOULA**
½ to 1 teaspoon smoked paprika, to taste
Juice of ½ to 1 lemon, to taste
½ bunch of cilantro
½ small bunch of flat-leaf parsley, leaves only
2 garlic cloves, peeled and roughly chopped
1-inch piece of fresh ginger,
   peeled and roughly chopped
½ red chile, seeded and roughly chopped
   (optional)
2 teaspoons ground cumin
Olive oil
Sea salt and freshly ground black pepper

1. Preheat the oven to 375°F.

2. Cut the sweet potatoes into chips about ¼ inch wide, leaving the skin on.

3. Put the chips into a large mixing bowl, drizzle over the olive oil, and season with salt and pepper. Toss well to make sure that each chip is coated with oil, then spread them in a single layer on two baking sheets. Put the sheets into the oven and bake for 15 minutes, then remove from the oven and turn the chips over. Return to the oven for an additional 7 to 10 minutes, until all the chips are golden.

4. While the chips are cooking, make the chermoula. Put all the ingredients except the oil into a food processor (starting with ½ teaspoon of smoked paprika and the juice of ½ lemon) and process until very finely chopped.

5. With the motor running, pour in enough olive oil (roughly 3 tablespoons) to bring the chermoula to a dipping consistency. Taste and adjust the amount of lemon juice and smoked paprika as necessary. Season with salt and pepper and blitz again to mix together.

6. Serve the hot chips with the chermoula dip. Any leftover chermoula can be stored covered in the fridge for up to a week.

**HOW TO USE CHERMOULA**
You can also use the chermoula to marinate meats and fish— just reduce the amount of oil in this recipe so the result is a stiffer paste.

| PER SERVING | |
| --- | --- |
| CALORIES | 318 |
| FAT (g) | 16.0 |
| SATURATED FAT (g) | 2.0 |
| CARBS (g) | 36.0 |
| SUGAR (g) | 19.0 |
| FIBER (g) | 3.0 |
| PROTEIN (g) | 7.0 |
| SODIUM (g) | 0.19 |

# HIGH-PROTEIN RECOVERY MEALS FOR THE EVENING AFTER

# CAULIFLOWER PIZZA

**SERVES 2 (MAKES 1 MEDIUM PIZZA)**

This is a very clever way of making pizza that little bit more healthy by cutting out refined carbohydrates and upping your veg intake at the same time. Add your favorite toppings, like ham, pepperoni, artichokes, olives, and jalapeños, and serve with a big green salad on the side. Kids love it, too, especially if you get them to put on their own toppings. They don't even suspect that it's cauliflower they're eating! And the mozzarella provides lots of calcium-rich protein to aid muscle recovery after an active day.

**FOR THE BASE**

1 medium cauliflower
½ teaspoon dried oregano
1 egg, beaten
⅓ cup grated Parmesan cheese
½ cup very finely chopped mozzarella cheese
Sea salt and freshly ground black pepper
Olive oil

**FOR THE TOPPING**

3 tablespoons tomato sauce
2 cremini mushrooms, sliced
1 thyme sprig, leaves only
⅔ cup thinly sliced mozzarella cheese
Sea salt and freshly ground black pepper

**CONTINUED ON PAGE 246**

| PER SERVING | |
| --- | --- |
| CALORIES | 405 |
| FAT (g) | 27.0 |
| SATURATED FAT (g) | 13.0 |
| CARBS (g) | 11.0 |
| SUGAR (g) | 8.0 |
| FIBER (g) | 6.0 |
| PROTEIN (g) | 26.0 |
| SODIUM (g) | 0.99 |

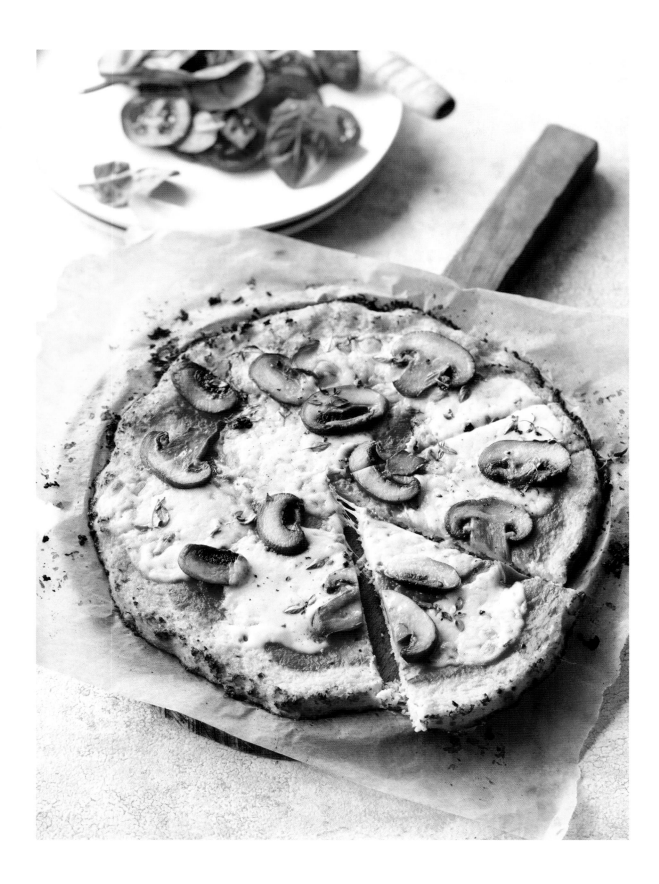

CONTINUED FROM PAGE 244

1. Preheat the oven to 425°F.

2. Break the cauliflower into florets and put them into a food processor, then blitz until they resemble breadcrumbs.

3. Put the cauliflower crumbs into a microwave-proof bowl and cover with plastic wrap, leaving a little gap. Cook on full power in the microwave for 6 minutes (see below). Remove and uncover, allowing the steam to escape and the crumbs to cool.

4. Place a baking sheet or pizza stone in the oven to heat.

5. Put the cooked cauliflower onto a clean tea towel or piece of cheesecloth. Draw the tea towel/cheesecloth up around the cauliflower and twist and squeeze until all the moisture has come out.

6. Put the cauliflower into a mixing bowl with the oregano, egg, cheeses, and a pinch of salt and pepper and mix together well.

7. Place a large piece of parchment paper on a cutting board and rub with a little olive oil. Turn out the cauliflower mixture onto the paper and shape it into a round pizza base about ⅓ inch thick. Rub the top of the pizza base with a little more olive oil.

8. Carefully lift the base, still on the paper, onto the preheated baking sheet or pizza stone, then bake in the oven for 8 to 12 minutes, until golden and crisp.

9. Remove from the oven and cover the top with the tomato sauce, using the back of a spoon to spread it out. Scatter with the sliced mushrooms and thyme leaves, then top with the sliced mozzarella and a sprinkle of salt and pepper.

10. Return the pizza to the oven for 5 to 7 minutes, until the cheese has melted and started to color. Slice and serve while hot.

---

**HOW TO COOK THE CAULIFLOWER CRUMBS**
If you don't have a microwave, steam, boil, or bake the crumbs for 5 to 6 minutes, until tender. The only difference is that you will have to work a bit harder to extract all the water in step 5.

# BARBECUED SPATCHCOCKED CORNISH GAME HENS WITH ROASTED CORN SALAD

**SERVES 4**

I love to barbecue, and over my many years of firing up the coals, I have learned that spatchcocking birds really is the best way to cook them evenly. It isn't hard to do (see below), but you can also get your butcher to do it for you. I have given instructions for oven-cooking, too, just in case the weather lets you down.

**FOR THE MARINADE**
1 tablespoon olive oil
1 small onion, peeled and finely diced
Sea salt
2 garlic cloves, peeled and finely chopped
1 teaspoon smoked paprika
2 tablespoons tomato purée
2 tablespoons maple syrup
2 teaspoons Worcestershire sauce
1 tablespoon balsamic vinegar
½ to 1 tablespoon soy sauce, to taste

**FOR THE HENS AND SALAD**
4 Cornish game hens, spatchcocked
4 ears corn on the cob, husks removed
Juice of 1 lime
1½ teaspoons chipotle paste
1 tablespoon maple syrup
2 tablespoons olive oil
Sea salt and freshly ground black pepper
1 red pepper, seeded and diced
1 small red onion, peeled and finely diced
3 to 4 cilantro sprigs, stems chopped, leaves reserved
1 (15-ounce) can black beans, adzuki beans, or pinto beans, drained and rinsed

**CONTINUED ON PAGE 249**

**HOW TO SPATCHCOCK A BIRD**
To spatchcock a cornish game hen, turn it breast side down with the legs toward you and, using sturdy kitchen scissors, cut along either side of the backbone and remove it. Open the bird out and turn it over so you can flatten it with your hand.

| PER SERVING | |
| --- | --- |
| CALORIES | 829 |
| FAT (g) | 47.0 |
| SATURATED FAT (g) | 11.0 |
| CARBS (g) | 34.0 |
| SUGAR (g) | 18.0 |
| FIBER (g) | 13.0 |
| PROTEIN (g) | 59.0 |
| SODIUM (g) | 1.16 |

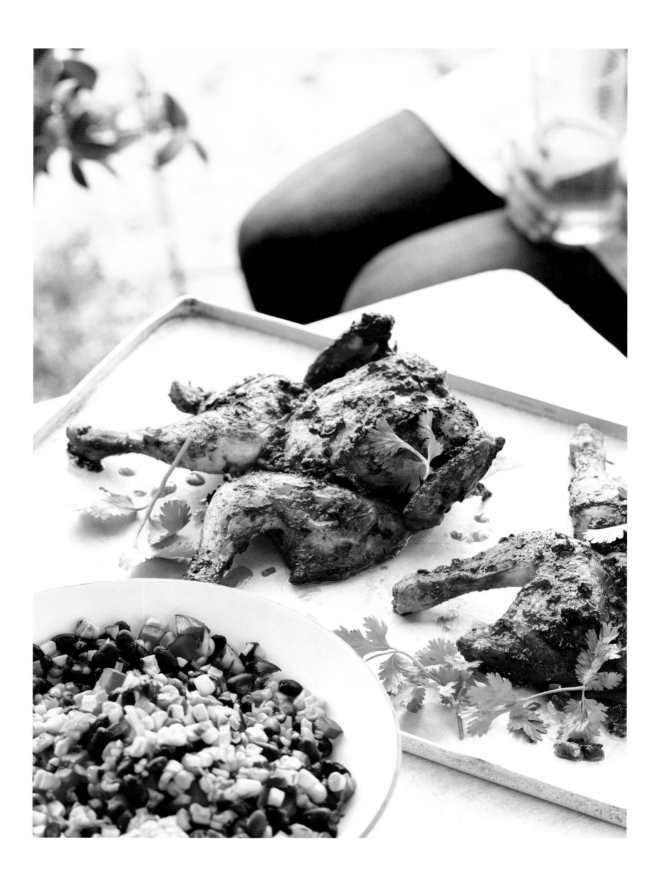

CONTINUED FROM PAGE 247

1. To make the marinade, place a small saucepan over medium heat and add the olive oil. Once hot, sauté the onion with a pinch of salt for 5 minutes, or until softened.

2. Add the garlic and continue to cook for 1 minute, then add the remaining marinade ingredients. Stir well and simmer gently for 5 to 6 minutes. Taste and adjust the seasoning as necessary, adding more soy sauce for a more savory flavor. Leave to cool.

3. When the marinade has cooled down, put the Cornish game hens into a container and pour over the marinade. Cover the dish with plastic wrap and put it into the fridge for at least an hour, or up to 2 days.

4. When ready to cook, light the grill or preheat the oven to 350°F and remove the birds from the fridge to let them come to room temperature.

5. To barbecue, when the coals are medium-hot, put the birds on the grill for 20 minutes, or until cooked through, turning after 10 minutes.

6. To oven-cook, put the marinated hens on a roasting sheet, breast side up, and into the oven. Roast for 30 to 35 minutes, until cooked through, basting occasionally. (If the extremities of the birds look like they might burn, cover with a piece of aluminum foil for the remainder of the cooking time.)

7. Meanwhile, heat a grill pan or grill until very hot and cook the corn on all sides until lightly charred. This will take 7 to 10 minutes. (To barbecue the corn, place the cobs on the grill before the chicken while the coals are still very hot.)

8. While the corn is cooking, put the lime juice, chipotle paste, maple syrup, olive oil and a pinch of salt and pepper into a jar with a tight-fitting lid and shake until combined.

9. Remove the kernels from the cobs by placing the cobs on their ends on a cutting board and running a sharp knife along the cobs. Put the kernels into a large mixing bowl.

10. Add the red pepper, red onion, cilantro stems, and beans and pour in the dressing. Toss well to make sure everything is coated, then taste and adjust the seasoning as necessary.

11. Once the birds are cooked, remove from the oven and leave to rest for 5 to 10 minutes. Sprinkle with the cilantro leaves and serve with the corn salad and lots of napkins!

# CELEBRATION SIDE OF SALMON WITH LEMON AND WASABI

**SERVES 6 TO 8**

This recipe is ideal for a post-race party—if you've got the energy to cook it, that is! It's very easy to put together, and the fish looks after itself once it's in the oven. The added bonus is that it is delicious served hot, warm, at room temperature, or even cold, so if you get distracted when it's out of the oven, it won't spoil. Better still, get someone else to cook it for you while you rest your aching muscles . . . Serve it with new potatoes, green salad, and lots of homemade mayonnaise.

1 (3½-pound) side of salmon, skin on, scaled and pinbones removed
Juice of 1½ lemons
2 teaspoons wasabi paste or powder
2 tablespoons Worcestershire sauce
2 tablespoons olive oil
Sea salt and freshly ground black pepper

**TO SERVE**
Arugula leaves
Lemon wedges

**1.** Preheat the oven to 400°F.

**2.** Place the side of salmon skin side down in a large roasting pan lined with parchment paper.

**3.** Mix together the lemon juice, wasabi, Worcestershire sauce, and olive oil until completely combined, then season with salt and pepper.

**4.** Pour the mixture over the salmon, making sure the sides of the salmon as well as the top have some of the marinade on them.

**5.** Put the pan into the oven and bake the salmon for 20 to 25 minutes, until just cooked through.

**6.** Remove from the oven and allow to rest for a few minutes. Scatter over some arugula leaves and serve with lemon wedges.

| PER SERVING | |
|---|---|
| CALORIES | 525 |
| FAT (g) | 34.0 |
| SATURATED FAT (g) | 6.0 |
| CARBS (g) | 2.0 |
| SUGAR (g) | 1.0 |
| FIBER (g) | 0.0 |
| PROTEIN (g) | 52.0 |
| SODIUM (g) | 0.44 |

**FEEDING A CROWD**
You can scale this recipe up if you are cooking for larger numbers. You should be able to fit two 3½-pound sides of salmon head-to-toe in a large roasting pan, or you can use two roasting pans and swap shelves halfway through cooking. Two sides of salmon should feed 12 to 15 people.

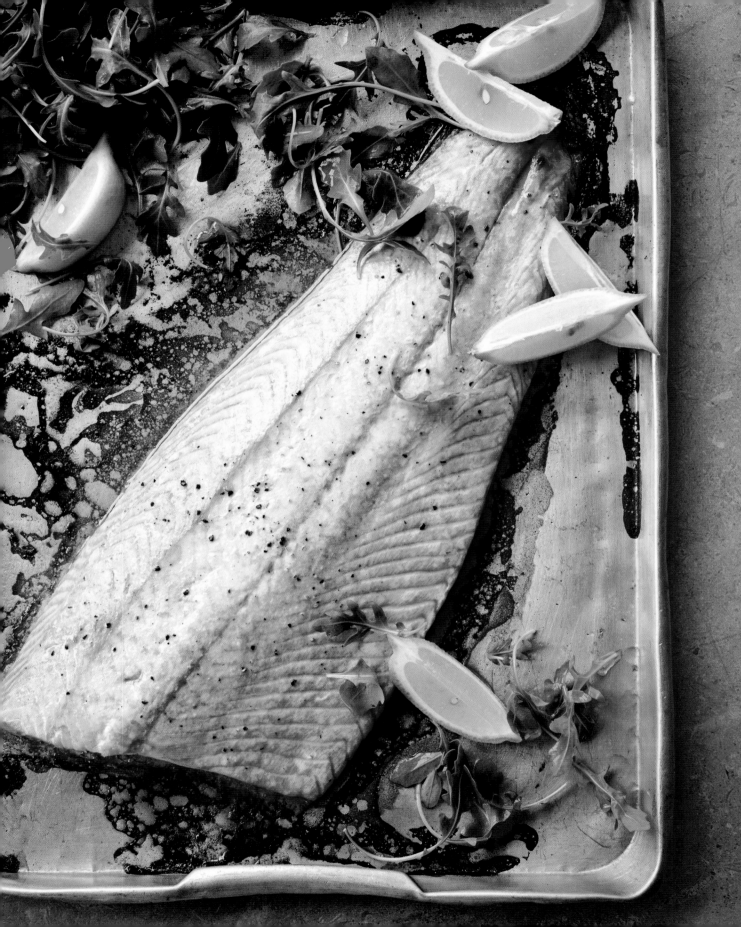

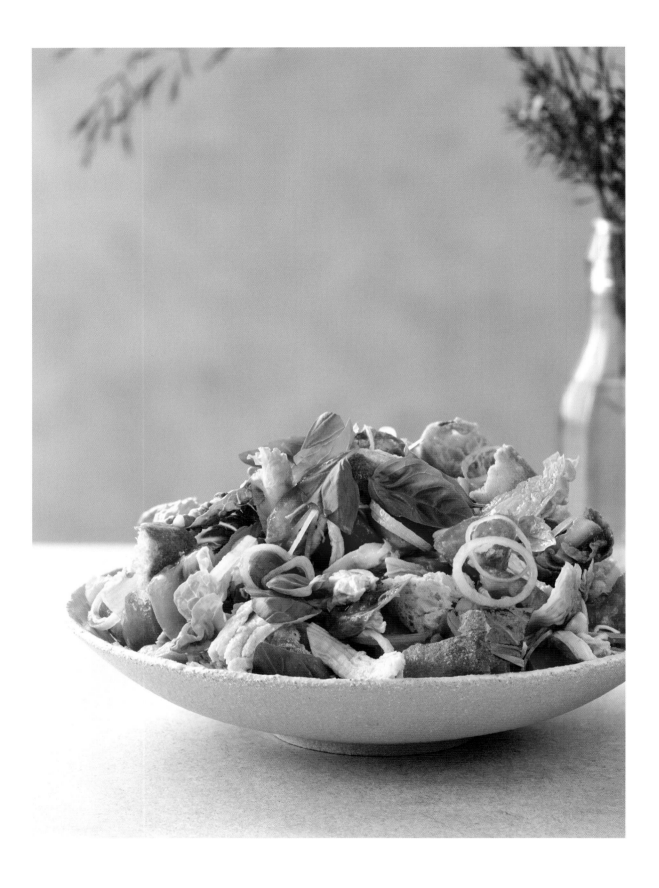

# PANZANELLA WITH POACHED CHICKEN

**SERVES 4**

Panzanella is an Italian bread and tomato salad with a strong anchovy dressing that will really liven up a simple poached chicken supper. As always when serving tomatoes, make sure you choose the ripest you can find, as they will have much more flavor and sweetness than unripe ones. Be careful not to boil the chicken breasts, and always leave them in the stock to cool because removing them from the liquid while hot will dry them out.

1 quart chicken stock
4 chicken breasts, skin removed
½ large ciabatta loaf
1½ tablespoons olive oil
2½ tablespoons red wine vinegar
2 large shallots, peeled and cut into thin rounds
1 rosemary sprig, leaves only
2 anchovy fillets, drained and finely chopped
4 large ripe tomatoes
3 Little Gem lettuces, leaves separated and washed
Sea salt and freshly ground black pepper
1 bunch of basil, leaves only

**1**. Preheat the oven to 350°F.

**2**. Put the chicken stock into a saucepan and bring to a boil. Add the chicken breasts, then reduce the heat to its lowest setting and cover with a lid. Cook the chicken for 10 minutes, then turn the heat off completely and leave the breasts to cool in the stock until you are ready to serve.

**3**. Cut the ciabatta into 1-inch chunks and scatter them over a baking sheet. Place in the oven and bake for 10 minutes, or until the bread has crisped up. Remove the sheet from the oven and leave to cool.

**4**. Pour the oil and red wine vinegar into a bowl and add the shallot rings, rosemary leaves, and chopped anchovies.

**5**. Place a sieve or colander over the bowl, then roughly chop the tomatoes into 12 large chunks per tomato and place in the colander. Roughly crush the tomatoes with the back of a wooden spoon to release some of their juice.

**6**. When ready to serve, tip the tomatoes from the sieve into a large serving bowl, then add the toasted bread and lettuce leaves.

**7**. Remove the chicken breasts from the stock and tear them into large chunks with a knife and fork, then add them to the salad bowl.

**8**. Whisk together the dressing mixture with the tomato juice, season with salt and pepper, and pour into the bowl. Toss everything together and sprinkle over the basil leaves before serving.

| PER SERVING | |
| --- | --- |
| CALORIES | 469 |
| FAT (g) | 14.0 |
| SATURATED FAT (g) | 3.0 |
| CARBS (g) | 30.0 |
| SUGAR (g) | 9.0 |
| FIBER (g) | 7.0 |
| PROTEIN (g) | 52.0 |
| SODIUM (g) | 1.52 |

# GARLIC AND PARSLEY GUINEA HEN STEW

**SERVES 4**

To me, this is the perfect evening meal after a winter race or heavy training session. It is so warming and restorative and full of the proteins and complex carbohydrates your body needs when it has pushed itself to the limit. Having spent time cooking in France, I really love guinea hen, especially cooked in this way, but you could easily make this with chicken, too. Note that guinea hen is a much leaner protein and therefore has less fat than chicken. Either way, you'll have a delicious home-cooked dinner.

1½ tablespoons olive oil
1 large guinea hen
Sea salt and freshly ground black pepper
1 onion, peeled and diced
1 carrot, diced
2 celery stalks, diced
1 bay leaf
½ small bunch of parsley, leaves picked
   and stems tied in a bundle with kitchen string
4 garlic cloves, peeled and sliced
½ cup dry sherry
2 cups chicken stock
¾ cup Puy lentils
Squeeze of lemon juice, or to taste

1. Preheat the oven to 350°F.

2. Place a large casserole dish with a lid over medium heat and add 1 tablespoon of the olive oil. Season the guinea hen with salt and pepper and, when the oil is hot, place breast side down in the casserole dish. Leave for 3 to 4 minutes to brown, then turn and continue browning until golden all over. Remove and set aside.

3. Add the remaining olive oil to the casserole and add the onion, carrot, celery, bay leaf, and parsley stems with a pinch of salt and pepper. Stir, cover with the lid, and cook for 6 to 8 minutes, until the onion is softened. Remove the lid, add the garlic, and cook for an additional 1 to 2 minutes, until aromatic and softened.

4. Add the sherry to deglaze the pan, scraping up any bits from the bottom, and allow to bubble for 2 minutes.

**CONTINUED ON PAGE 256**

| PER SERVING | |
| --- | --- |
| CALORIES | 500 |
| FAT (g) | 16.0 |
| SATURATED FAT (g) | 4.0 |
| CARBS (g) | 23.0 |
| SUGAR (g) | 4.0 |
| FIBER (g) | 7.0 |
| PROTEIN (g) | 54.0 |
| SODIUM (g) | 0.67 |

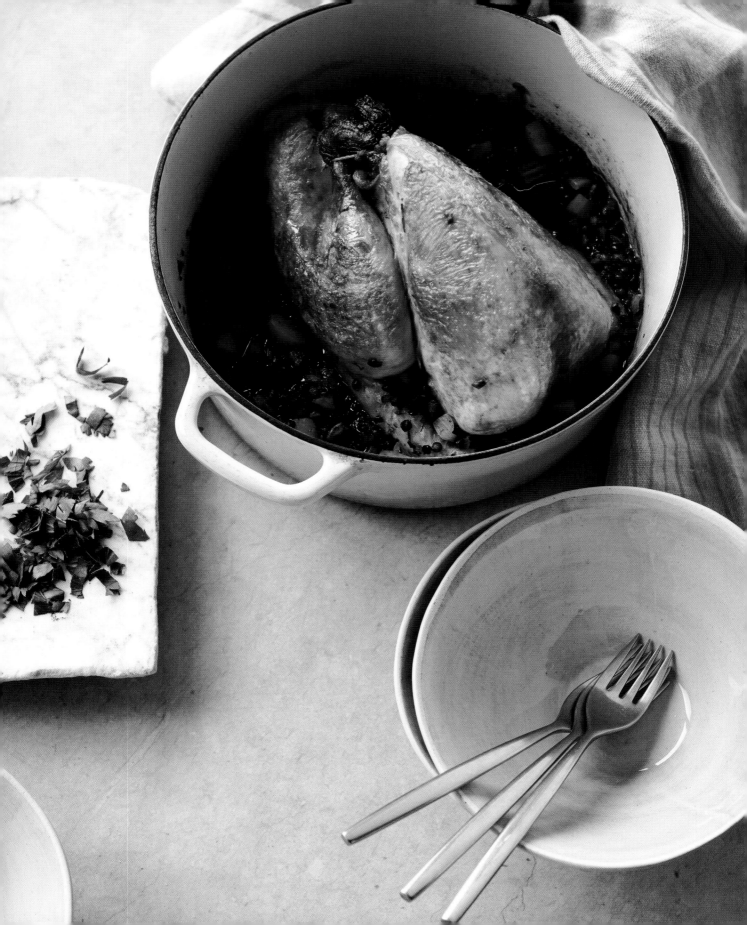

CONTINUED FROM PAGE 254

**5**. Add the chicken stock and the lentils and stir, then put the guinea hen, breast side up, back into the casserole dish, pushing it down into the lentils so that the liquid and the lentils rise up around the bird.

**6**. Put the lid on, transfer to the oven, and bake for 50 minutes. Remove the lid and give the lentils a stir, then put back into the oven and cook for an additional 10 minutes uncovered, to color the skin on the breast a little more.

**7**. Remove from the oven and take the guinea hen out of the casserole. Put it on a board to rest for 5 minutes.

**8**. Meanwhile, give the lentils a stir and taste. Add a squeeze of lemon and a little salt and pepper if needed, and taste again to check the seasoning. Remove the parsley stems and bay leaf.

**9**. Roughly chop the parsley leaves, add to the dish, and stir through.

**10.** Cut up the guinea hen (see below) and put the pieces back into the casserole dish with the lentils. Pour any juices that run off while carving into the lentils.

**11.** Bring the casserole dish to the table for people to help themselves, and serve with seasonal green vegetables.

**HOW TO CUT UP COOKED POULTRY**
Cut through the skin that joins the legs to the breast and pull the legs away from the body until they come free at the joint. Using a very sharp knife, cut down between the thigh and the drumstick to separate them. To remove the breasts, run the knife along the breastbone, pulling the breast away as you cut.

# SPICED KOFTAS WITH BULGUR WHEAT SALAD

SERVES 4

The flavors of the Middle East and North Africa converge in this protein-rich dish. It is a particularly good choice for a recovery meal because everything can be made in advance, with only the broiling of the koftas to be done on the spot, leaving you to enjoy a well-deserved rest before tucking into a delicious restorative feast.

2 tablespoons olive oil
2 small red onions, peeled and diced
1 garlic clove, peeled and diced
1 (15-ounce) can cannellini beans, drained and rinsed
1 (14.5-ounce) can chopped tomatoes
1 to 2 teaspoons harissa paste, to taste
Sea salt and freshly ground black pepper
2 cups chicken or vegetable stock
1¾ cups dried bulgur wheat
4 ounces lean ground lamb
6 ounces lean ground turkey
1 egg

⅔ cup fresh breadcrumbs
1½ teaspoons ground cinnamon
1½ teaspoons ground cumin
½ bunch of parsley, roughly chopped
½ bunch of mint, leaves roughly chopped
Juice of 1 lemon

**TO SERVE**
Flatbreads
0% fat Greek yogurt

**CONTINUED ON PAGE 259**

| PER SERVING | |
| --- | --- |
| CALORIES | 561 |
| FAT (g) | 12.0 |
| SATURATED FAT (g) | 3.0 |
| CARBS (g) | 67.0 |
| SUGAR (g) | 8.0 |
| FIBER (g) | 16.0 |
| PROTEIN (g) | 37.0 |
| SODIUM (g) | 1.04 |

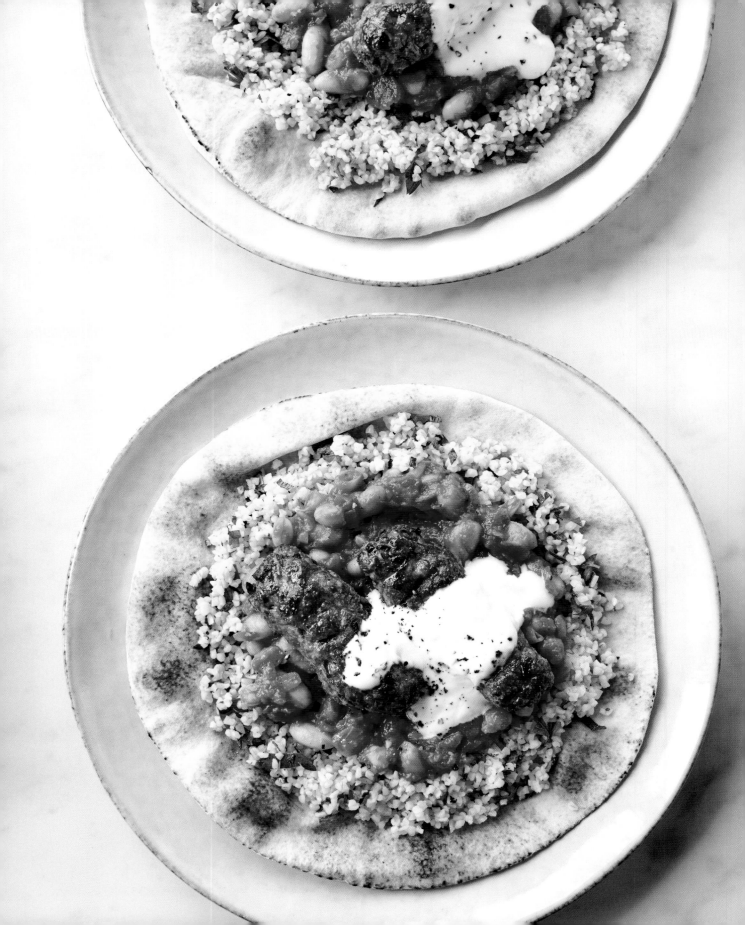

CONTINUED FROM PAGE 257

**1.** Place a saucepan over medium-high heat and add 1 tablespoon of the olive oil. When hot, add half the diced onion and the garlic and cook for 5 minutes. Add the cannellini beans and chopped tomatoes along with half a can of water. Bring the liquid to a boil, then reduce to a simmer and cook for 10 minutes.

**2.** Remove the pan from the heat, stir in the harissa paste, and season with a little salt and pepper.

**3.** Bring the chicken stock to a boil and tip the bulgur wheat into a large bowl. When the stock is boiling, pour it over the bulgur, cover with plastic wrap, and leave to sit for a minimum of 10 minutes.

**4.** Meanwhile, using clean hands, mix the two ground meats with the egg, breadcrumbs, cinnamon, cumin, the remaining diced red onion, and a good pinch of salt and pepper. Work the mixture until it comes together, then mold into 8 small sausage shapes.

**5.** Heat the broiler to high and, when hot, broil the koftas for 8 to 10 minutes, turning a few times. Make sure they are fully cooked through by cutting into a thick kofta to check that the meat is no longer pink in the middle.

**6.** Turn the broiler off and leave the meat to rest in the warmth of the broiler.

**7.** Remove the plastic wrap from the bulgur wheat, pour in the remaining tablespoon of olive oil, and fluff the grains with a fork. Add the parsley, mint, and lemon juice, season with a good pinch of salt and pepper, and stir.

**8.** Serve the koftas with the beans, bulgur salad, flatbread, and a big dollop of Greek yogurt.

# FLANK STEAK WITH ROSEMARY CHIMICHURRI

**SERVES 4**

Because flank steak is less tender than other cuts, it is often marinated or slow-cooked. When it is cooked on a grill pan like this, it is vital to keep the cooking time down so that it is served medium-rare and then to carve it against the grain to keep it from being chewy. This can get very smoky, so turn the exhaust fan to max and open the windows. It's ideal for barbecuing in the great outdoors, too.

½ bunch of parsley, finely chopped
½ small bunch of oregano, leaves finely chopped
3 garlic cloves, peeled and crushed
2 rosemary sprigs, leaves finely chopped
1 red chile, seeded and finely chopped
2½ tablespoons red wine vinegar
2 tablespoons canola
Sea salt and freshly ground black pepper
2¼ pounds flank steak
4 portobello mushrooms, brushed clean
  and cut into thick slices
12 whole cherry tomatoes on the vine
Watercress, to serve

1. Mix together the parsley, oregano, garlic, rosemary, chile, red wine vinegar, and a third of the oil. Season with a little salt and pepper, then leave to infuse for approximately 2 hours.

2. When ready to cook, heat a large grill pan over high heat.

3. Brush the steak on both sides with the remaining oil, then, when the griddle is smoking hot, carefully put it onto the pan and cook for 4 minutes on each side. Remove the steak, wrap in aluminum foil, and leave to rest.

4. Put the sliced mushrooms on the grill pan in a single layer and cook for 2 minutes on each side. Take the mushrooms off the pan, then add the tomatoes and cook for approximately 2 minutes as well.

5. Carve the steak against the grain into long, thin slices and arrange the slices on a serving platter. Drizzle with a generous amount of chimichurri and serve with the mushrooms, tomatoes, and watercress.

| PER SERVING | |
| --- | --- |
| CALORIES | 554 |
| FAT (g) | 32.0 |
| SATURATED FAT (g) | 10.0 |
| CARBS (g) | 4.0 |
| SUGAR (g) | 4.0 |
| FIBER (g) | 4.0 |
| PROTEIN (g) | 60.0 |
| SODIUM (g) | 0.45 |

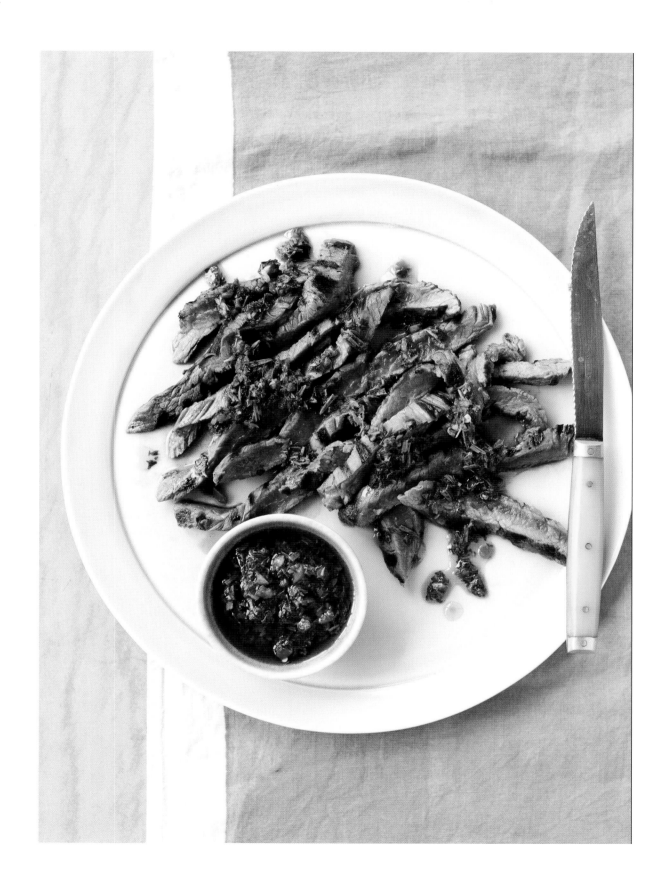

# HIGH-ENERGY SNACKS AND WELL-DESERVED TREATS

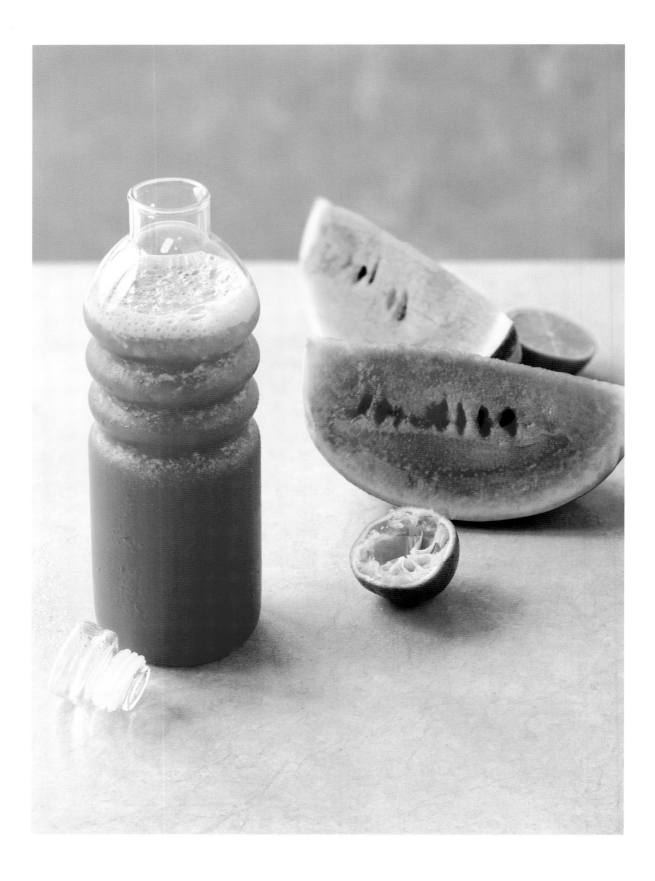

# WATERMELON COOLER

**SERVES 6**

What you drink before, during, and after exercise is just as important as what you eat, and this easy juice provides excellent hydration as well as instant energy without any free sugars. The pinch of salt isn't essential, but it helps replenish the body's sodium levels, which are seriously depleted by sweating over a long period of time.

2 pounds seeded watermelon flesh, cut into chunks
Juice of 1 lime
Pinch of salt

1. Put the watermelon chunks into a blender and blitz until smooth. Add the lime juice and a pinch of salt and blend again.

2. Add 2 handfuls of ice and blend once more or until the ice is broken up. If the mixture is very thick, blend in ½ cup of cold water.

3. Serve in glasses with extra ice cubes or pour into your water bottle to take with you.

**VARIATIONS**
You can alter the flavor slightly by adding herbs or a pinch of cayenne. Basil works well, as does mint.

| PER SERVING | |
| --- | --- |
| CALORIES | 56 |
| FAT (g) | 0.3 |
| SATURATED FAT (g) | 0.0 |
| CARBS (g) | 12.0 |
| SUGAR (g) | 10.0 |
| FIBER (g) | 1.0 |
| PROTEIN (g) | 1.0 |
| SODIUM (g) | 0.9 |

# PITA CHIPS WITH RED PEPPER DIP

**SERVES 4**

Making your own pita chips is both healthier and cheaper than buying store-bought chips when you're having dips. They are the perfect accompaniment for snacks like the Minted Baba Ghanoush on page 95 and the Smoky Cannellini Bean Hummus on page 94 and are an easy way to add more carbs to soups and salads when you need them. The dip is very versatile, too—it's delicious with seafood such as shrimp or grilled squid and is also great on pasta.

4 large whole-wheat pita breads
1 garlic clove, peeled and crushed
½ teaspoon Italian seasoning
2 tablespoons olive oil
Sea salt

**FOR THE RED PEPPER DIP**
12 ounces jarred roasted red peppers, drained
1½ teaspoons sherry vinegar
⅔ cup slivered almonds
2 tablespoons olive oil
Sea salt and freshly ground black pepper

1. Preheat the oven to 350°F.

2. Cut each pita bread into 8 triangles, then divide each triangle into 2 thinner triangles and place them in a single layer on two baking sheets.

3. Mix together the crushed garlic, Italian seasoning, and olive oil. Brush each side of the triangles with a little of the mixture and sprinkle with a pinch of salt. Put the sheets into the oven and bake for 3 to 4 minutes, then turn the triangles over, removing any thinner pieces that are already crisp. Return the sheets to the oven and bake for an additional 2 to 3 minutes, until all the triangles are golden brown and crisp. Remove from the oven and leave to cool.

4. For the red pepper dip, put all the ingredients into a food processor and blitz until smooth, then season with salt and pepper. If the consistency is a bit thick, add a tablespoon of water and blitz again.

5. Serve the pita chips and some fresh crudités with the dip as a great on-the-go lunch or a snack for sharing with friends. Any leftover dip can be stored covered in the fridge for up to 3 days.

| PER SERVING | |
| --- | --- |
| CALORIES | 386 |
| FAT (g) | 22.0 |
| SATURATED FAT (g) | 3.0 |
| CARBS (g) | 32.0 |
| SUGAR (g) | 3.0 |
| FIBER (g) | 4.0 |
| PROTEIN (g) | 12.0 |
| SODIUM (g) | 1.95 |

**HOW TO STORE PITA CHIPS**
The pita chips can be stored in an airtight container for up to a week. If they need crisping up before eating, put them into an oven preheated to 300°F for 2 to 5 minutes.

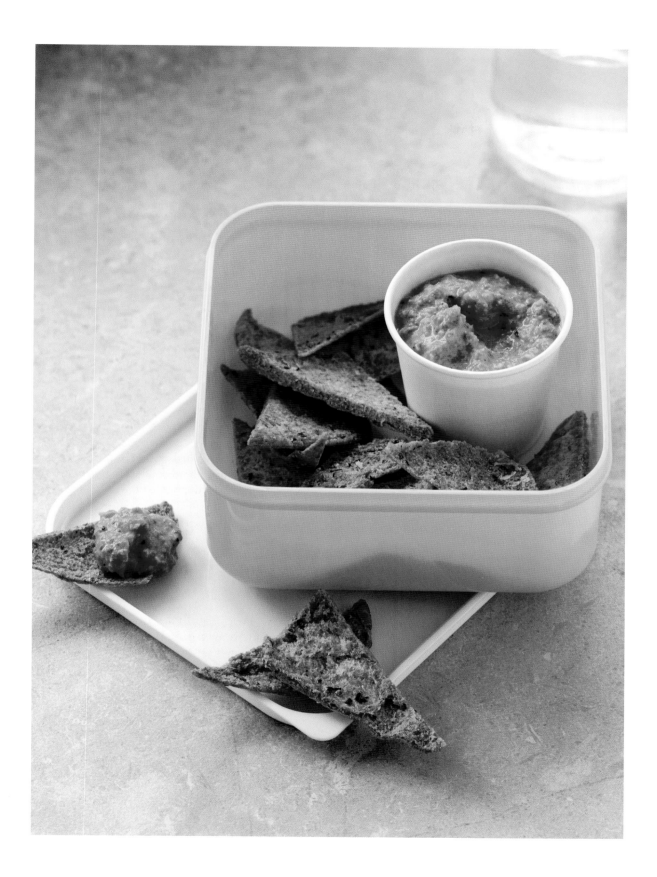

# SEED AND NUT "GRANOLA" BARS
**MAKES 18 BARS**

Granola bars are my go-to snacks when I'm training for a triathlon. They're easy to make, perfect for carrying around, and they give me everything I need to be able to perform at my absolute best. The dates act as the glue that binds everything together, but you can vary the other ingredients depending on what you like or have in the pantry. These are also good for camping trips, picnics, and packed lunches.

1⅓ cups dates, pitted
2 tablespoons nut butter, such as peanut, cashew, or almond butter
2 tablespoons coconut oil
1¼ cups rolled oats
¾ cup almonds
½ cup Brazil nuts
2 tablespoons mixed seeds, such as sunflower, pumpkin, and flaxseeds
2½ cups puffed brown rice (optional)

1. Place the dates in a food processor with ¼ cup of hot water and process until smooth. If the mixture is a bit lumpy, add hot water 1 tablespoon at a time, processing between additions until you have a smooth paste.

2. Add the nut butter and coconut oil and process until combined, then add the oats, almonds, and Brazil nuts and pulse briefly to mix through but not break down completely.

3. Gently stir in the mixed seeds and puffed rice, if using, by hand.

4. Line a baking pan (approximately 11 × 7 inches) with waxed paper and pour the mixture into the pan. Flatten the surface until roughly level.

5. Cover with plastic wrap and put into the fridge to chill until completely firm (about an hour).

6. Cut into squares or bar shapes, and keep in the fridge for up to a week.

| PER BAR | |
| --- | --- |
| CALORIES | 139 |
| FAT (g) | 8.0 |
| SATURATED FAT (g) | 2.0 |
| CARBS (g) | 12.0 |
| SUGAR (g) | 8.0 |
| FIBER (g) | 2.0 |
| PROTEIN (g) | 3.0 |
| SODIUM (g) | 0.01 |

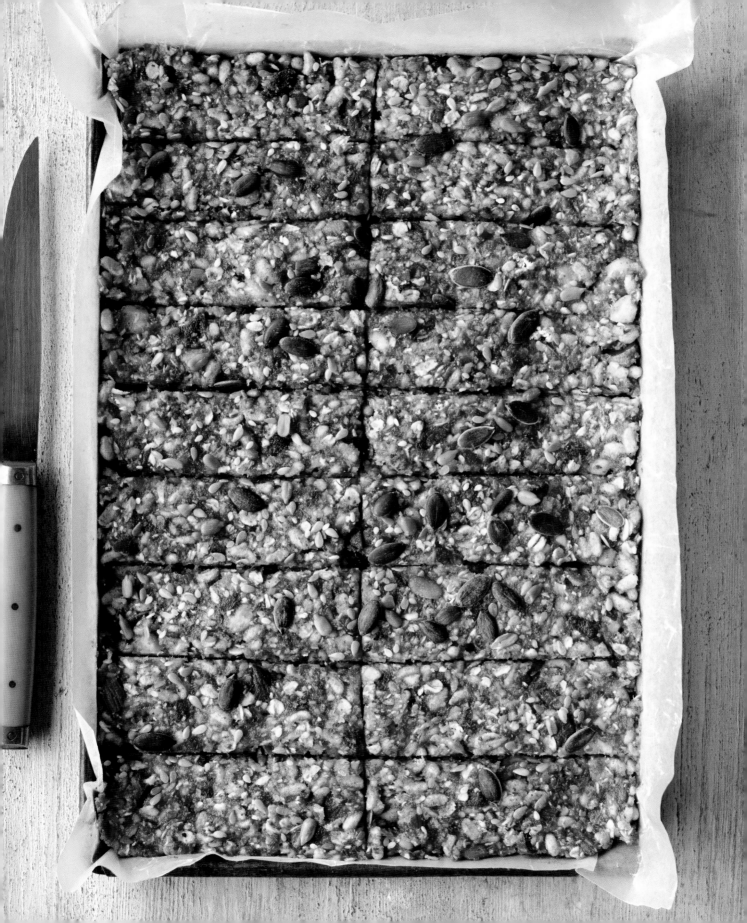

# RAW CHOCOLATE MILK SHAKE

**SERVES 4**

If you get a craving for a chocolate milk shake, make it as natural as possible by blitzing up your own with almond milk, cacao nibs, and dates. Yes, it's really sweet, but the fiber in the dates and the natural fats in the cacao powder mean the energy is slow-releasing and won't wreak havoc on your blood sugar levels after consuming. Swap the almond milk for cow's milk if you need extra protein after a tough workout or competition.

1 quart unsweetened almond milk
½ cup cacao powder
8 to 12 dates, pitted
Maple syrup (optional)

1. Put the almond milk, cacao powder, and dates into a blender and blitz until smooth.

2. Taste and add a little maple syrup, if needed.

3. Add a handful of ice cubes to the milk shake and blend again to chill completely.

4. Pour into four glasses and serve with a straw.

| PER SERVING | |
| --- | --- |
| CALORIES | 154 |
| FAT (g) | 6.0 |
| SATURATED FAT (g) | 2.0 |
| CARBS (g) | 17.0 |
| SUGAR (g) | 14.0 |
| FIBER (g) | 7.0 |
| PROTEIN (g) | 6.0 |
| SODIUM (g) | 0.33 |

**VARIATION**
You can also add banana and nut butter to this milk shake.

# GRANOLA ENERGY BITES

**MAKES 14 BITES**

These oat, fruit, and nut energy balls are the equivalent of eating a bowl of granola in a couple of bites. They are full of easy-access energy when you need it most, and are brilliant for when you don't have time for breakfast or for a quick boost before a workout or run. We always have a version of these or the Raw Choco Treats (page 273) in the fridge so everyone in the family can help themselves when they need to.

⅓ cup unsweetened peanut butter, smooth or crunchy
3 tablespoons runny honey
1½ cups rolled oats
1 cup raisins
½ cup walnuts, very finely chopped

1. Mix together the peanut butter and honey in a large mixing bowl until combined. Pour in the oats, raisins, and finely chopped walnuts and mix really well, until everything is coated in the peanut butter honey mixture.

2. Place the mixture in the fridge for 20 minutes to firm up a little.

3. Once firm, remove from the fridge and, using your hands, form the mixture into balls about 1½ inches wide, squeezing the mixture together to make it stick. Place the balls on a baking sheet and chill in the fridge for at least an hour to set.

4. Transfer to an airtight container and store in the fridge, where they will keep for 1 to 2 weeks.

**HOW TO MAKE GRANOLA COOKIES**
To turn these bites into crisp cookies, put the balls onto a baking sheet lined with parchment paper and press into flat circles. Put the sheet into an oven preheated to 325°F and bake for 10 to 12 minutes, until golden and crisp on the outside and chewy on the inside.

| PER ENERGY BITE | |
| --- | --- |
| CALORIES | 150 |
| FAT (g) | 7.0 |
| SATURATED FAT (g) | 1.0 |
| CARBS (g) | 17.0 |
| SUGAR (g) | 11.0 |
| FIBER (g) | 2.0 |
| PROTEIN (g) | 4.0 |
| SODIUM (g) | 0.08 |

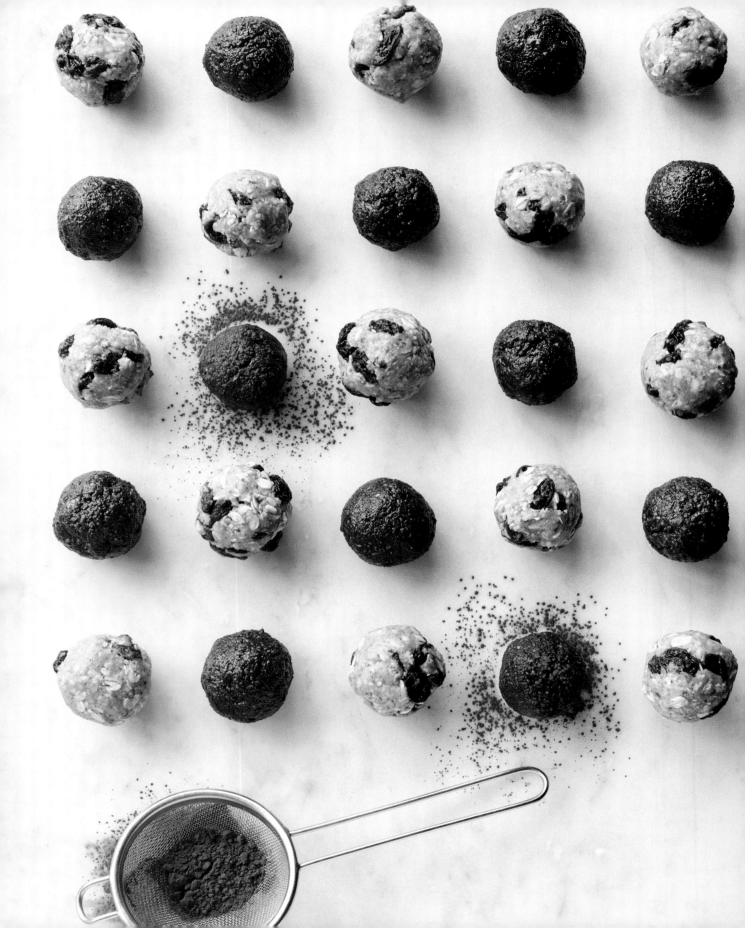

# RAW CHOCO TREATS

**MAKES 14 TREATS**

Tana has given me her secret recipe for these incredible chocolate snacks, which are also known as "bliss balls." You can add any nuts or seeds that you like or roll them in desiccated coconut for a bit of crunch. They make a really good pre-exercise snack as well as a general energy boost in the middle of a busy day.

½ cup pitted dates
2 tablespoons coconut oil
1 tablespoon almond butter
¾ cup almonds
3 tablespoons cacao powder, plus a little for dusting

**1.** Put the dates and coconut oil into a food processor and process until a smooth paste has formed.

**2.** Add the almond butter and process to mix, then add the almonds and process again until they are finely chopped.

**3.** Finally, add the cacao powder and process until the mixture starts to stick together and all the ingredients are finely chopped.

**4.** Using a teaspoon, take 1 heaping spoonful of the mixture and roll it between your hands into a ball. Place on a plate or baking sheet and repeat with the remaining mixture. Dust with a little extra cacao powder, then cover the balls with plastic wrap and put into the fridge to firm up for at least 2 hours.

**5.** Once firm, transfer them to an airtight container and keep them in the fridge for up to 2 weeks.

**HOW TO MAKE AHEAD**
Make a big batch of these balls and freeze the spares. They taste delicious straight from the freezer, or can be defrosted in the fridge until ready to eat.

| PER TREAT | |
| --- | --- |
| CALORIES | 78 |
| FAT (g) | 6.0 |
| SATURATED FAT (g) | 2.0 |
| CARBS (g) | 4.0 |
| SUGAR (g) | 4.0 |
| FIBER (g) | 1.0 |
| PROTEIN (g) | 2.0 |
| SODIUM (g) | 0.01 |

# FIG BARS
**MAKES 16 BARS**

It would be impossible to calculate how many fig bars I have eaten in my lifetime . . . Let's just agree that it's a lot! It started when my mum used to put them in my lunchbox when I was a kid and now, forty years later, they are one of my favorite training snacks. For me, a homemade snack in the middle of a triathlon gives me more than just a physical energy boost, it lifts my spirits in a way that an isotonic gel or store-bought granola bar never could.

2 cups dried figs, stems trimmed and roughly chopped
2 cups whole-wheat flour, plus a little extra for dusting
1 teaspoon baking powder
⅓ cup coconut oil
¼ teaspoon salt
½ teaspoon ground cinnamon
1 egg
⅓ cup 2% reduced-fat milk, plus a little extra for brushing
2 pinches of turbinado sugar

1. Put the chopped figs into a saucepan with 1 cup water and bring to a boil over medium–high heat. Cover with a lid, reduce the heat to low, and simmer for 15 minutes, or until the figs are very soft and the water is absorbed. Keep an eye on the pan to make sure it doesn't cook dry.

2. Remove the pan from the heat and, using the back of a wooden spoon, press on the figs to break them up a bit. Tip the figs into a bowl and leave them to cool completely.

3. Put the flour, baking powder, coconut oil, salt, and ground cinnamon into a food processor and blitz until the ingredients are fully incorporated.

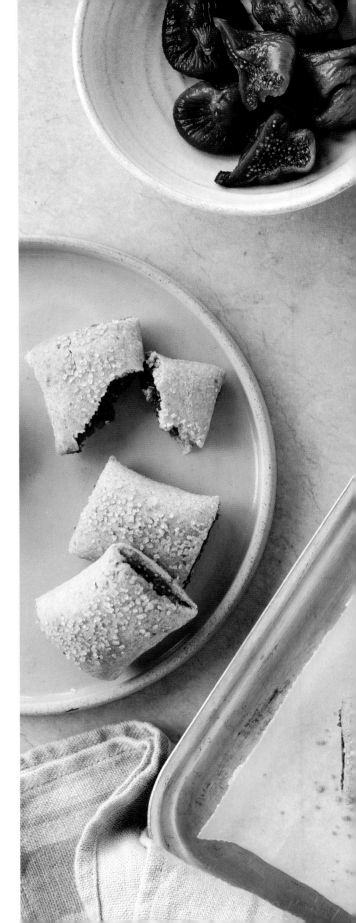

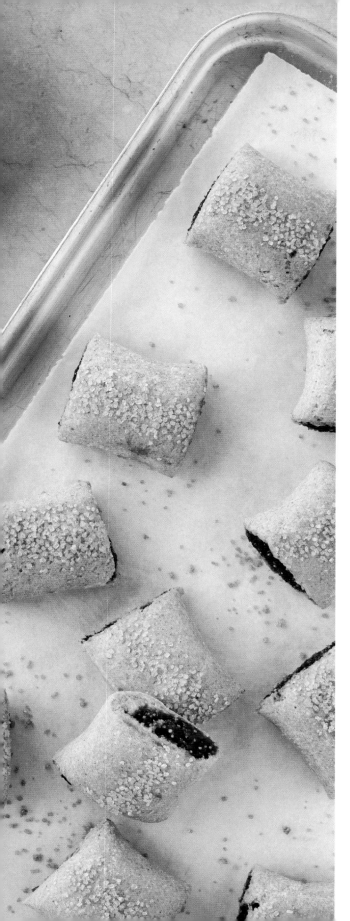

**4**. Add the egg and milk and pulse until the pastry comes together.

**5**. Tip the pastry onto a clean work surface and knead for 30 seconds, then wrap in plastic wrap and leave to rest for 20 minutes.

**6**. Meanwhile, preheat the oven to 400°F.

**7**. Unwrap the pastry and cut it into 2 equal-size pieces. Dust a clean surface with a little flour, then roll out the first half into a rectangle roughly 16 × 16 inches that's about ⅛ inch thick.

**8**. Spoon half of the fig mixture in a line across the middle of the rectangle. Roll one side of the pastry over the other, gently pushing to join the seam. Trim any excess pastry from all the seams, then repeat the process with the other piece of pastry.

**9**. Brush the rolls with milk, then sprinkle with sugar and cut each one into 8 equal-size pieces. Place the pieces onto a baking sheet lined with parchment paper, then place in the oven and bake for 15 minutes, or until lightly browned on top.

**10**. Remove the sheet from the oven and allow the fig bars to cool completely before eating.

---

**HOW TO MAKE THE PASTRY**
This pastry really needs to be made in a food processor to incorporate the coconut oil. It can be done by hand, but it takes a very long time!

| PER FIG BAR | |
| --- | --- |
| CALORIES | 150 |
| FAT (g) | 5.0 |
| SATURATED FAT (g) | 4.0 |
| CARBS (g) | 23.0 |
| SUGAR (g) | 9.0 |
| FIBER (g) | 3.0 |
| PROTEIN (g) | 3.0 |
| SODIUM (g) | 0.07 |

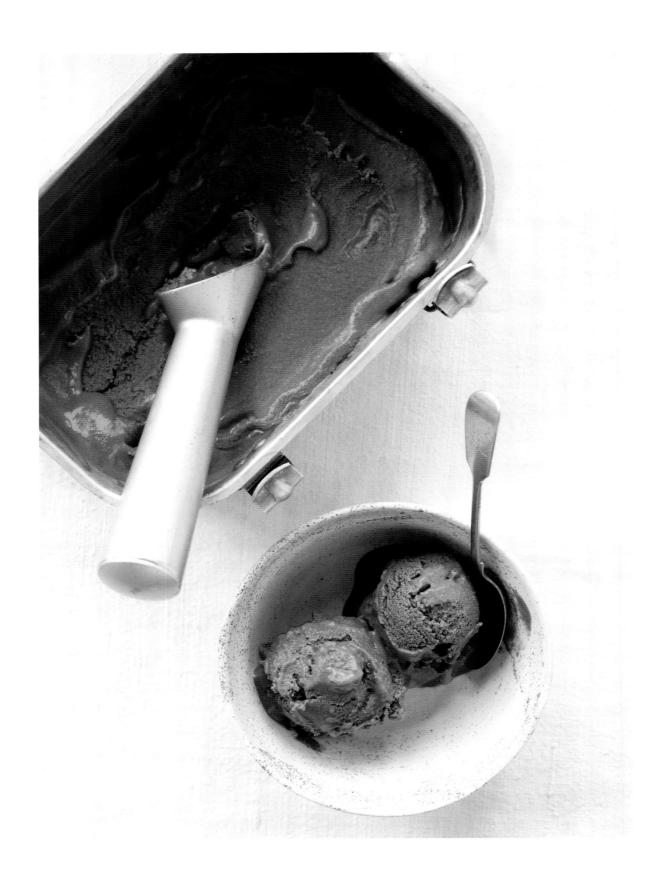

# PEANUT BUTTER AND CHOCOLATE ICE CREAM

**SERVES 6**

This is a variation of the incredibly simple Banana "Ice Cream" on page 180, with added peanut butter to provide a post-exercise protein hit for tired muscles. The coconut milk makes it even more creamy, and can also restore some of the vital nutrients lost when taking part in strenuous training. It's extremely indulgent but really great when you've earned it.

1 (14-ounce) can coconut milk
1 large ripe banana, cut into chunks and frozen for at least 4 hours
3 tablespoons peanut butter, smooth or chunky
2 tablespoons cacao powder
Honey or maple syrup (optional)

1. Put the coconut milk and banana into a food processor and process until smooth, occasionally scraping down the sides.

2. Add the peanut butter and cacao powder and blend until well mixed. Taste and sweeten with honey or maple syrup, if necessary.

3. Pour into a freezer-proof container with a lid and put into the freezer for 2 to 4 hours, until almost set.

4. Remove from the freezer and process again, then put back into the container and freeze until set. This should result in a smoother ice cream with fewer ice crystals.

5. To serve, remove from the freezer 20 to 30 minutes before serving to allow for easy scooping.

**VARIATION**
If you prefer not to use coconut milk, you can make this by simply blending 4 chopped frozen bananas with the peanut butter and the cacao until smooth, then freezing.

| PER SERVING | |
| --- | --- |
| CALORIES | 190 |
| FAT (g) | 16.0 |
| SATURATED FAT (g) | 11.0 |
| CARBS (g) | 7.0 |
| SUGAR (g) | 5.0 |
| FIBER (g) | 2.0 |
| PROTEIN (g) | 4.0 |
| SODIUM (g) | 0.07 |

# CHEESECAKE IN A JAM JAR

**SERVES 4**

This is a really indulgent treat for when it's all over . . . It's almost as naughty as a regular cheesecake, but the almonds in the base and the Greek yogurt mixed into the topping mean that it's a more nourishing version than the classic; it's full of protein, calcium, and vitamins to support your muscles and bones after exertion. Putting this in jam jars makes it very portable, but if you are staying at home, you can use glasses instead.

**FOR THE BASE**

1⅓ cups almonds, skins on
3 tablespoons coconut oil
2 tablespoons coconut sugar

**FOR THE TOPPING**

1 cup low-fat cream cheese, at room temperature
1½ cups plain Greek yogurt
1 to 2 tablespoons coconut sugar, maple syrup, or runny honey, to taste
1 tablespoon lemon juice
1 tablespoon vanilla extract
Pinch of salt
1¼ cups frozen blueberries, defrosted

**1.** Toast the almonds in a dry skillet over medium heat for 3 to 4 minutes, until they smell nutty and toasted. Leave to cool slightly.

**2.** Pour the toasted almonds into a food processor and blitz until finely chopped. Add the coconut oil and coconut sugar and process until completely incorporated.

**3.** Divide the mixture among four small jam jars and press down to make a firm base. Place the jars in the fridge to firm up while you make the topping.

**4.** Put the cream cheese and yogurt into a mixing bowl and beat together with a wooden spoon. Once mixed, add 1 tablespoon of the coconut sugar with the lemon juice, vanilla, and a pinch of salt. Mix again and taste, adding the remaining sugar if needed.

**5.** Stir half the blueberries into the topping and roughly mix so that they aren't completely broken up but instead give a swirling pattern to the mixture.

**6.** Remove the jam jars from the fridge and divide the topping mixture among them, filling each one until there is a ¾-inch gap at the top. Tap the bottom of the jars gently on the work surface to level out the filling.

**7.** Divide the remaining blueberries among the jars, making sure you don't overfill them if you plan to put the lids on for transportation.

**8.** Return the jars to the fridge and chill for at least an hour to firm up.

**9.** Serve the cheesecakes straight from the fridge, or put them into an insulated bag to take with you on a picnic.

| PER SERVING | |
| --- | --- |
| CALORIES | 638 |
| FAT (g) | 46.0 |
| SATURATED FAT (g) | 16.0 |
| CARBS (g) | 28.0 |
| SUGAR (g) | 22.0 |
| FIBER (g) | 2.0 |
| PROTEIN (g) | 24.0 |
| SODIUM (g) | 0.55 |

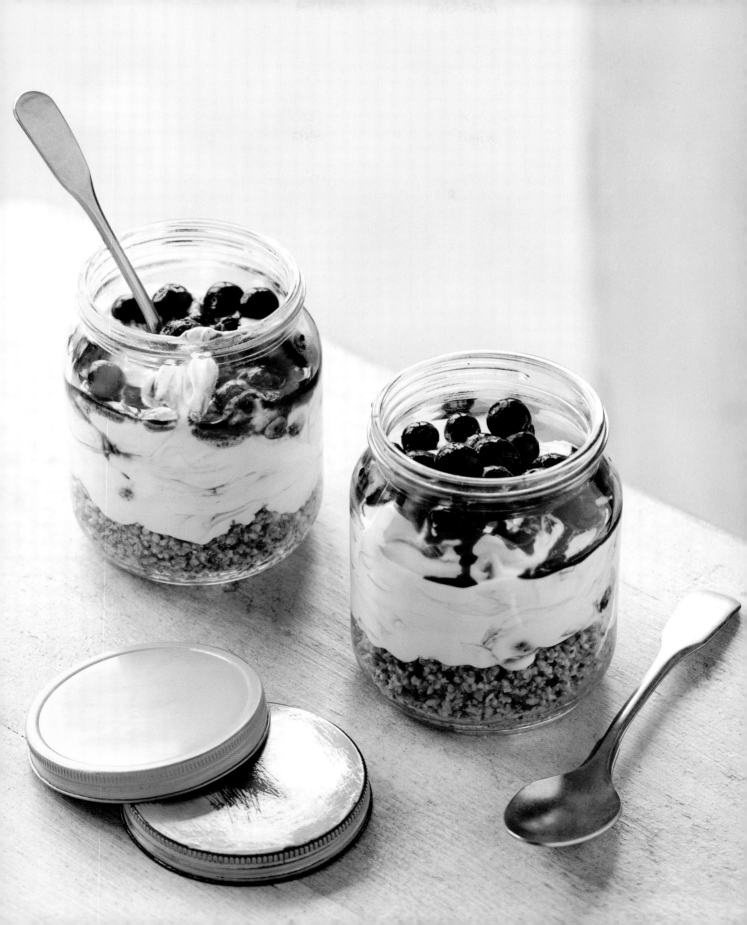

# AZTEC HOT CHOCOLATE

**MAKES 4 SMALL CUPS**

This is a short, dark, rich hot chocolate shot rather than a big milky mugful. Similar to an espresso, it packs a powerful punch and makes a really warming treat after a winter workout or race. Dark chocolate with a high cocoa content has lots of nutritional benefits, such as improving circulation, reducing "bad" cholesterol, and protecting skin and eyes, so you can happily indulge in this without any guilt!

3½ ounces dark chocolate
  (at least 70% cocoa solids), grated
1 teaspoon vanilla extract
Pinch of freshly grated nutmeg
½ teaspoon cayenne pepper (optional)
1 to 2 tablespoons runny honey or maple syrup, to taste
2 cinnamon sticks, halved

**1.** Heat 2 cups of water in a small pan until hot but not boiling. Add the chocolate and whisk over medium–low heat until well combined and thick.

**2.** Stir in the vanilla extract, nutmeg, and cayenne, if using, then sweeten to taste with the honey.

**3**. Gently heat for an additional 5 to 8 minutes, to allow the flavors to infuse. Whisk occasionally and be careful not to let the mixture boil.

**4.** Serve in espresso cups or small glasses with half a cinnamon stick to flavor and stir.

| PER SERVING | |
|---|---|
| CALORIES | 165 |
| FAT (g) | 11.0 |
| SATURATED FAT (g) | 6.0 |
| CARBS (g) | 13.0 |
| SUGAR (g) | 10.0 |
| FIBER (g) | 3.0 |
| PROTEIN (g) | 2.0 |
| SODIUM (g) | 0.05 |

# INDEX

# ACKNOWLEDGMENTS

Putting a cookbook together is a bit like running a marathon relay race—many talented people hold the baton at different stages and each of them, in turn, helps the project to cross the finishing line. I therefore need to say thank you to all the great runners in my team . . .

Thank you so much to the amazing folk at Hodder & Stoughton for their vision, commitment, and encouragement throughout: editorial director Nicky Ross, project editor Natalie Bradley, art director Alasdair Oliver, production manager Claudette Morris, marketing manager Catriona Horne, and publicity director Louise Swannell. It's a dream team!

I am also very lucky to be supported by a great lineup behind the scenes. Many thanks to Camilla Stoddart and Annie Lee for their help with the words and to Anna Horsburgh and Rob Allison for their help with the food. An extra special thank-you must go to nutritionist Kerry Torrens, who kept us all on track with a firm and patient hand—her knowledge and passion for her subject is hugely inspiring and she's a pleasure to work with.

The stunning pictures in the book are thanks to the winning combination of art director James Edgar, photographer Jamie Orlando Smith, food stylist Phil Mundy, and prop stylist Olivia Wardle. Thank you all.

Thanks also to the mighty Justin Mandel in the States and Rachel Ferguson in the UK for organizing my busy life and making sure I am where I am supposed to be every day. I couldn't make the distance without you.

I am also ever grateful to all of my trainers and the fellow cycle enthusiasts and triathletes that I've met who keep me pushing every day.

And last, thank you to my incredible family, who keep me going at the twenty-fifth mile and always inspire me to give my best. Tana, Megan, Jack, Holly, and Tilly—you are my favorite training partners and the motivation for everything I do.